CONTENTS

ABBREVIATIONS

AC	anterior chamber
ACG	angle closure glaucoma
ACTH	adreno cortico trophic hormone
AH	aqueous humour
AT	applanation tonometry
BP	blood pressure
BRVO	branch retinal vein occlusion
CCF	carotico-cavernous fistula
CF	central field, counting fingers
CNS	central nervous system
CRAO	central retinal artery occlusion
CRVO	central retinal vein occlusion
CSG	chronic simple glaucoma
CSR	central serous retinopathy
CT	cover test
CT Scan	computed tomography
D	dioptre
DCG	dacryocystography
DCR	dacryocystorhinostomy
EC	extracapsular
EOG	electro-oculogram
ERG	electro-retinogram
ESR	erythrocyte sedimentation rate
EUA	examination under anaesthesia
FFA	fluorescein fundus angiogram
G	guttae
GA	general anaesthesia
Hg	mercury
HM	hand movements
I & C	incision and curettage
IC	intracapsular
ICP	intracranial pressure
IM	intramuscular
IOFB	intraocular foreign body
ION	ischaemic optic neuropathy
IOP	intraocular pressure

Abbreviations

KCS	keratoconjunctivitis sicca
KP	keratic precipitates
LA	local anaesthesia
LGB	lateral geniculate body
NPL	no perception of light
OA	optic atrophy
Oc	occulentum
OKN	optokinetic nystagmus
PCT	prism cover test
PH	pinhole
PL	perception of light
RB	rose bengal
RBN	retrobulbar neuritis
RD	retinal detachment
RLF	retrolental fibroplasia
SC	subconjunctival
SG	Sheridan Gardner
SO	superior oblique
USG	ultrasonography
VA	visual acuity
VER	visual evoked response

ACKNOWLEDGEMENTS

We express our thanks to Miss Sheila Graham SRN OND for suggesting that we write this book and for helping us to plan its format. All the diagrams have been drawn by Mr Peter Jack. He has earned our admiration and gratitude for the way in which he has transformed our preliminary sketches into such informative drawings that complement the text so well. The book would not be so extensively illustrated had it not been for the generosity of Merck Sharp & Dohme and two patients, who wish to remain anonymous. Miss Ruth Malpas SRN OND, our Nursing Tutor kindly read an early draft and we are most grateful to her for the amendments she proposed.

We are greatly indebted to Miss Mina Yuille for compiling the index and to Miss O'Callaghan SRN OND for writing the Foreword. Miss Sara Hipwell's skill in preparing the typescript is beyond praise.

Finally, we acknowledge the patience and encouragement shown to us by our publisher throughout the preparation of the book.

FOREWORD

Most nurses are involved from time-to-time in the care of patients with eye problems or visual handicap. Obtaining the necessary background information to support and teach these patients has often proved a frustrating task, even for specialised nurses. They have struggled with the complexity of advanced texts, or experienced disappointment at the paucity of detail in over-simplified volumes.

Here, at last, is a book that presents medical and surgical ophthalmology in straightforward terms to meet the needs of the specialist Ophthalmic Nurse, and of nurses in hospital and community settings. The authors have produced a succinct text, generously illustrated with bold diagrams which are an invaluable aid to understanding. The emphasis throughout is on principles, and nurses will find this approach most helpful when planning and implementing patient care. The book is in two parts, the first giving background information and outlining the principles of ophthalmology, the second dealing with specific disorders and treatments.

In Part One, the chapters on anatomy, physiology and optics are sufficiently detailed to satisfy the basic requirements of the Ophthalmic Nursing Board's Courses. The systematic headings and stated principles for history taking and examination of the eye are valuable guides. There is a brief introduction to the work of theatres, the out-patient department and casualty. The chapter on microbiology outlines the organisms that may be found in and around the eye, and discusses the principles of taking and dealing with specimens. There is an excellent chapter on ophthalmic pharmacology, providing an overview of preparations in current use, with summarising tables for easy reference.

Part Two covers a wide range of eye disorders, including ocular manifestations of systemic diseases. Of necessity, some are mentioned only briefly, while the commoner problems are described in greater detail. Here again, the illustrations are first-class, especially the diagrams depicting steps in surgical procedures. The text is simple, with specialised terminology kept to a minimum. For example, nurses who have found squint terminology confusing, will enjoy the refreshingly clear presentation of the subject, which is further enhanced by the inclusion of an illustrative case history. The final chapter outlines the facilities available for the registered blind, and gives useful hints on assisting the visually impaired in the Eye Hospital. The list of abbreviations and the glossary will prove helpful to those meeting the language of ophthalmology for the first time.

Foreword

In summary, this concise, well-illustrated and very readable book lays a broad foundation upon which the specialist Ophthalmic Nurse can build. Indeed, all nurses will find it a valuable source of up-to-date ophthalmic information, assisting them to plan care and offer appropriate advice to patients.

B.O'Callaghan (Miss), BA, SRN, OND, RNT
Director of Nursing Studies — Moorfields Eye Hospital, London
Director of Examinations — Ophthalmic Nursing Board

PREFACE

Eyes are of crucial importance. When we damage them, or notice something wrong with them, most of us become extremely anxious and fear that we may go blind.

A nurse who knows about the eye can be of tremendous help to many patients. If she is working in a Casualty Department or in a factory, she may save someone from blindness by treating a chemical burn promptly and effectively. If she is working with the elderly, many of them will have problems with their eyes and they will benefit greatly from talking to someone who understands their condition. The nurse working in general practice or in the community service may well have the opportunity of identifying children with eye disorders and play a role in ensuring that they receive the appropriate treatment.

The idea that we should write this book was suggested to us by Miss Sheila Graham, who worked as a Ward Sister, initially at Moorfields Eye Hospital and, later, at the Southampton Eye Hospital. She pointed out to us that there was a need for a book that related both the medical and surgical aspects of eye disorders to the work of a nurse. Having gained experience in this field over the past few years by working with nurses studying for the Ophthalmic Nursing Diploma, we have taken her advice.

Our aim has been to cater for the nurse who initially knows nothing about the eye. We set out to show, first, how the eye works and, then, go on to describe what may go wrong with it. This leads naturally to treatment. We have tried to emphasise underlying principles for they dictate the rationale of treatment (which itself may vary according to the fashion of the moment). We have used simple diagrams liberally to complement the text for we feel that even a simple illustration can often put across information more readily than many words.

We hope that this approach will lead to more nurses working in many different fields learning about the eye and so preparing themselves to help the patients who come under their care.

PART ONE

BACKGROUND AND GENERAL PRINCIPLES

1 THE EYE IN BRIEF

Sight is for most people their most treasured sense. Our ability to see normally depends upon both of our eyes working properly and the many parts of the brain which are involved in vision functioning satisfactorily.

The eye itself is rather like a camera. Essentially the light entering the eye is brought to a focus, by means of a lens, on to a light sensitive membrane — the retina (Figure 1.1). The retina in the eye is comparable to the film in a camera. The amount of light reaching the retina is controlled by the size of the pupil, just as the aperture in the diaphragm of the camera controls the amount of light reaching the film. Similarly, the focusing of both the eye and a camera may be varied so that objects either in the far distance or close to can be brought into sharp focus on the retina or film respectively.

Figure 1.1: The Globe

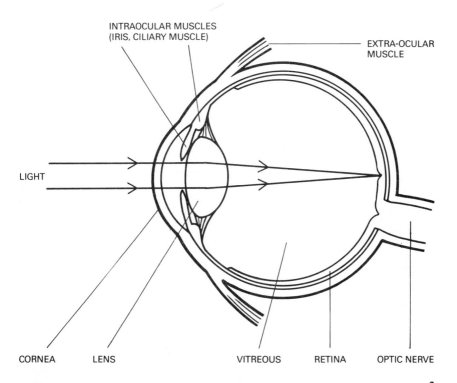

INTRAOCULAR MUSCLES
(IRIS, CILIARY MUSCLE)

EXTRA-OCULAR MUSCLE

LIGHT

CORNEA   LENS   VITREOUS   RETINA   OPTIC NERVE

The structures lying in front of the retina must necessarily be completely transparent for otherwise some light will not reach the retina and vision will be impaired. Opacities in the so-called optical media are a frequent cause of poor sight.

When light reaches the retina, various complex chemical and electrical changes are induced in special cells (rods and cones) which lead to electrical impulses leaving the eye, via the optic nerve, to travel right to the back of the brain along the optic pathways. It is in the occipital lobes that the impulses are converted into the sensation of sight. The long course of the optic pathways through the brain largely explains why vision is affected in so many cerebral disorders.

The eyes have a wide excursion which contributes to our enjoying a wide field of vision. The alignment of the eyes must be perfect for otherwise double vision will probably ensue. The control of eye movement is extremely complex, involving several parts of the brain, and the actions of the six muscles attached to each eye are normally co-ordinated in a very precise way.

In subsequent chapters the way in which we see is explained in greater detail and, later, many of the disorders that may impair vision are described. In due course the reader may feel amazed not that some of us sometimes see badly, but, rather, that any of us ever see as well as we do.

2 ANATOMY AND PHYSIOLOGY

This chapter deals with the structure (anatomy) of the various parts of the eye, together with that of the tissues closely related to the eye (the adnexae). Those anatomical features that have particular clinical relevance are stressed. Linked to this description of the anatomy is a consideration of the normal functioning of each part (i.e., its physiology). By considering jointly the anatomy and the physiology of each structure the wonderful way in which each individual part of the eye is constructed in order to fulfil a particular role becomes apparent.

Orbit

The orbits are two roughly conical cavities that house the eyes, which lie either side of the nasal cavity (Figure 2.1). The apices of the cones lie posteriorly. The cones are flattened on four sides so that each orbit is described as having a roof and a floor and medial and lateral walls. These walls are extremely thin, particularly in young children, so that they are easily fractured and often prove an inadequate barrier to infection spreading from the adjacent paranasal air sinuses. In contrast, the opening of the orbit, the base of the cone, is surrounded by an approximately square margin which is composed of relatively thick bone. It is the combination of the eye being deeply set in the orbit and the strength of the orbital margin that prevents the eye being injured more frequently than it is.

The orbit is surrounded on three sides by paranasal air sinuses. The exception is temporally. These sinuses, which are cavities within the bones of the skull are lined with mucus membrane and they communicate with the nasal cavity. Hence they are prone to become infected, causing sinusitis. The main benefit of our having such sinuses is that the weight of our head is greatly reduced.

The frontal sinus, above, separates the orbit from the anterior cranial cavity, in which lies the frontal lobe clothed in its covering of pia arachnoid and dura mater. An injury through the roof of the orbit with, perhaps a stick, may therefore result in meningitis or a brain abscess. On the medial side lie the ethmoidal air cells, in front, and the sphenoidal air cells behind. The former are a common source of organisms causing orbital cellutitis. Below, lies the large maxillary sinus — the antrum. A fracture of the floor of the orbit may allow some of the contents of the orbit to prolapse down into the antrum (a 'blow-out' fracture, chapter 9). In the reverse direction, an antral carcinoma may spread upwards and consequently displace the eye both upwards and forwards. In either event, the infra-orbital nerve, which supplies sensory branches to the cheek and which travels along the floor, may be damaged.

The orbit is essentially a bony box, which is open anteriorly. This anterior

5

Figure 2.1: The Orbits and Paranasal Air Sinuses

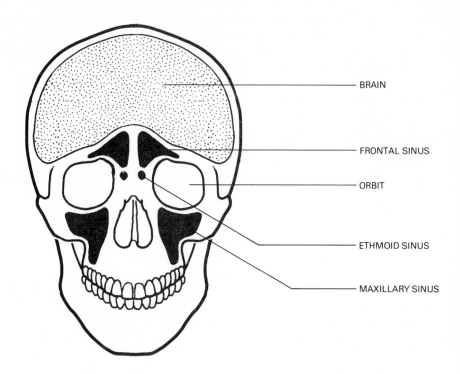

BRAIN

FRONTAL SINUS

ORBIT

ETHMOID SINUS

MAXILLARY SINUS

opening is largely closed off by the lids and the orbital septum, which is a sheet of fascia that runs from the periphery of the tarsal plates, that lie within the lids, to the orbital margin. Any space-occupying lesion in the orbit causes displacement of the eye, and because of the bony confines of the orbit, the major displacement is necessarily forwards. Convention has it that when one eye comes forwards (for example, due to an optic nerve tumour), the term proptosis is used. When both eyes come forward (for example, in dysthyroid eye disease) the term exophthalmos is employed.

At the back of the orbit lies the optic foramen, which transmits the optic nerve and the ophthalmic artery, with the accompanying sympathetic nerve fibres. The superior orbital fissure transmits branches of the ophthalmic division of the trigeminal (fifth cranial) nerve, together with the trochlear (fourth) and the abducent (sixth) nerves, which supply the superior oblique and lateral rectus muscles respectively. Orbital veins travel back through the inferior orbital fissure.

In the front of the orbit the lacrimal gland lies in a hollow above and laterally. The lacrimal sac lies in a fossa below and medially.

Many of the contents of the orbit, particularly the extraocular muscles, are invested with fascia (Tenon's capsule). The space between the many structures packed into the orbit is filled up with fat.

Lids

The lids close off the orbits anteriorly. They thus play an important part in the protection of the eyes. Their blinking action sweeps the tear film downwards and medially across the cornea and helps to remove any foreign bodies that may alight on the eye.

Figure 2.2: Cross-sections of the Eyelids

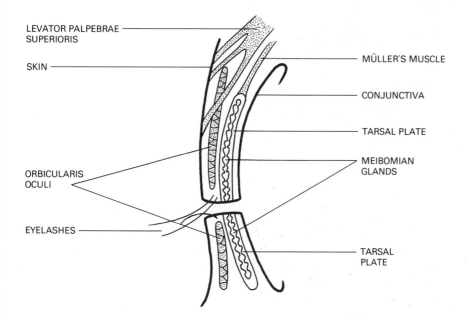

The lids consist, in essence, of modified flaps of skin in which are set the tarsal plates (Figure 2.2). These plates stiffen the lids to some extent. The form of the upper tarsal plate becomes clearly apparent when the lid is everted. The position of the tarsal plates is stabilised by medial and lateral palpebral ligaments which extend from the plates to the adjacent orbital margin (Figure 2.3). In each tarsal plate is a series of 40 or so Meibomian glands which are arranged vertically. (Hence a vertical incision is made in incising and curetting Meibomian cysts.) These glands produce the outer oily layer of the tear film which helps to minimise the evaporation of tears. The posterior aspect of each tarsal plate is covered with conjunctiva.

Into the upper border of each upper tarsal plate is inserted Müller's muscle (supplied by the sympathetic nervous system). A lesion of the sympathetic pathways causes a slight droop of the upper lid (ptosis). The major elevator of the upper lid is the levator palpebrae superioris (Figure 2.3). It sends fibres into the

Figure 2.3: Muscles of the Eyelids

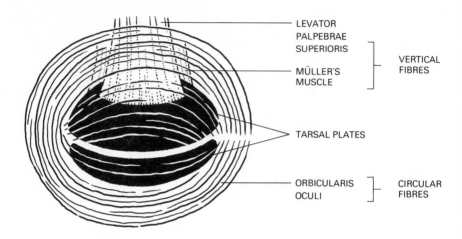

anterior part of the upper tarsal plate and also fibres that pass forward into the skin of the lid. The levator is supplied by the oculomotor (third cranial) nerve. A complete third nerve palsy causes (among other things) a complete ptosis.

In front of the levator tendon and the tarsal plates lies the plane in which the various blood vessels and nerves run. In front of this plane is the orbicularis oculi muscle which is, in a sense, a sphincter. Its contraction closes the lids. Because its innervation is from its deep surface, the local anaesthetic given prior to surgery on the orbicularis muscle (for example, operations for the correction of entropion or ectropion) should be injected deep into the muscle. Slips of the muscle pass in front of and behind the lacrimal sac, so creating a 'lacrimal pump' when blinking occurs. (The tiresome watering of the eye that occurs following a facial palsy, is, in part at least, due to loss of this pumping action.)

Anterior to the orbicularis, which is supplied by the facial (seventh cranial) nerve, lies the skin. The hairs are modified at the margin of the lid to form two rows of lashes. There are associated sweat and sebaceous glands.

Lacrimal Apparatus (Figure 2.4)

The lacrimal gland is located in the upper outer quadrant of the orbit in the lacrimal groove, behind the rim of the orbit. It secretes tears into the upper fornix. By their constant blinking movements the eyelids distribute the tears evenly over the cornea and encourage their flow towards the medial canthus. Tears drain through the puncta and canaliculi (especially the lower canaliculus) into the lacrimal sac and so on through the naso-lacrimal duct into the nose.

Normally the eye is covered by a thin film of tears which consists of three

Figure 2.4: The Lacrimal Apparatus

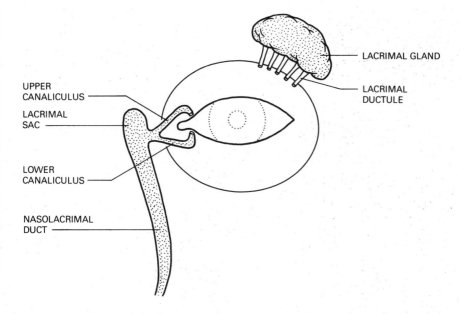

LACRIMAL GLAND

LACRIMAL
DUCTULE

UPPER
CANALICULUS

LACRIMAL
SAC

LOWER
CANALICULUS

NASOLACRIMAL
DUCT

Figure 2.5: The Pre-corneal Tear Film

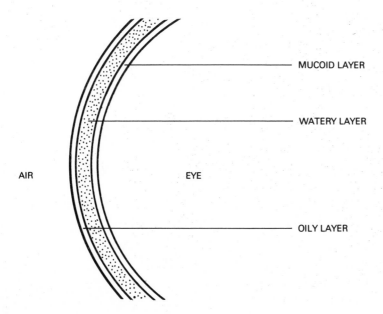

MUCOID LAYER

WATERY LAYER

AIR

EYE

OILY LAYER

layers (Figure 2.5). The inner mucus layer, which acts as a wetting agent, is derived from the conjunctival glands. The central watery layer is produced by the lacrimal glands. The outer oily layer, which minimises evaporation of the tears, comes from the Meibomian glands.

Tears bring oxygen to the cornea and help to wash away foreign bodies from the surface of the eye. Tear deficiency may be followed by serious complications (see chapter 11).

Conjunctiva (Figure 2.6)

The conjunctiva is a membrane which lines the back of the eyelids and covers the front of the eye apart from the cornea. The conjunctival and corneal epithelia though different in appearance, form a continuous layer over the front of the eye. The conjunctiva covering the lids is known as the palpebral part and that covering the anterior sclera and the tendons of the recti as the bulbar conjunctiva. The palpebral and bulbar conjunctivae join one another at the fornices. Together they form the conjunctival sac. Foreign bodies can enter the conjunctival sac through the palpebral aperture but cannot get behind the eye. Thus a contact lens can never be lost behind the eye. (See chapter 3.)

Figure 2.6: The Conjunctival Sac

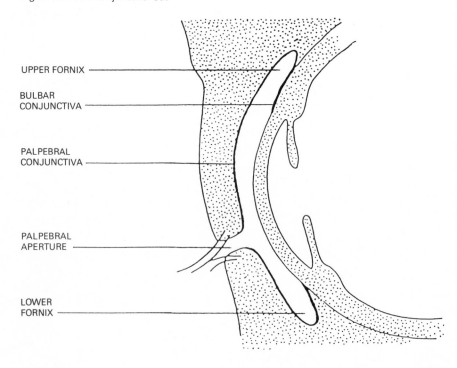

UPPER FORNIX

BULBAR
CONJUNCTIVA

PALPEBRAL
CONJUNCTIVA

PALPEBRAL
APERTURE

LOWER
FORNIX

At the inner canthus there is a knob of modified skin — the caruncle. It may have hairs sprouting from it. Lateral to it lies the plica, the remnant of the third eyelid or nictitating membrane of many animals.

Cornea (Figure 2.7)

The cornea is the clear 'window' at the front of the eye. It is usually 11.5mm in diameter. It is only 1.0mm thick in the periphery and it is even thinner centrally (0.5mm).

The cornea has five layers (Figure 2.8). The outermost layer, the epithelium, is easily rubbed off the underlying Bowman's membrane, causing a painful abrasion (chapter 23). Bowman's membrane does not regenerate so that if it is damaged, as it often is by foreign bodies lodging on the cornea, a scar will result.

The central layer, the stroma, contributes most to the thickness of the cornea. It consists of bundles of collagen fibres which are arranged in a particular pattern. This pattern is dependent upon the stroma being kept relatively dehydrated. If fluid accumulates then the stroma becomes opaque and the patient's vision worsens.

It is the innermost layer, the endothelium, set on Descemet's membrane that is responsible for pumping excess water out of the stroma. This 'endothelial pump' is necessary to keep the cornea transparent. The 'pump' is readily deranged by trauma or infection.

There are no blood vessels in the normal cornea. This means that it is free of antibodies. Consequently a graft set in an avascular cornea is unlikely to be rejected (chapter 13). The cornea is abundantly supplied with nerves from both the short and the long ciliary nerves so that any corneal disorder tends to be extremely painful.

Sclera

The sclera is the tough, white, outer coat of the eye. It merges with the cornea at the limbus. It is about 1.0mm thick throughout most of its extent. However, just behind the insertion of the tendons of the rectus muscles, it is a good deal thinner (0.4mm). It is just in this particularly thin part of the sclera that the surgeon needs to place his sutures when he recesses a muscle during squint surgery.

The sclera is elastic in children but it becomes inelastic with increasing age. Thus, if the intraocular pressure becomes raised in a baby, as in infantile glaucoma, then the eye becomes enlarged. However, the eye of an elderly patient with glaucoma remains unchanged in size.

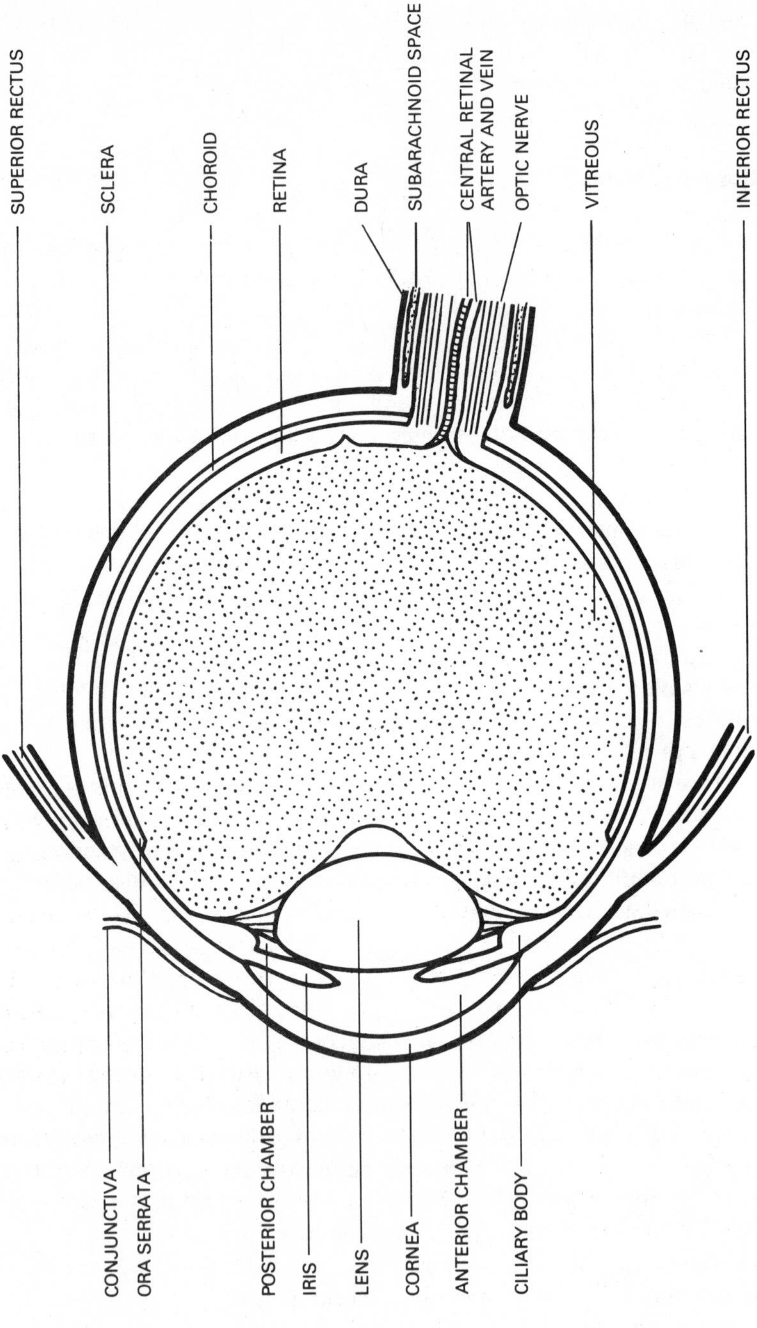

Figure 2.7: The Globe

SUPERIOR RECTUS

SCLERA

CHOROID

RETINA

DURA

SUBARACHNOID SPACE

CENTRAL RETINAL ARTERY AND VEIN

OPTIC NERVE

VITREOUS

INFERIOR RECTUS

CONJUNCTIVA

ORA SERRATA

POSTERIOR CHAMBER

IRIS

LENS

CORNEA

ANTERIOR CHAMBER

CILIARY BODY

Figure 2.8: The Cornea

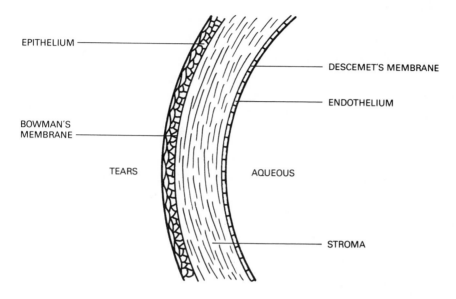

EPITHELIUM

DESCEMET'S MEMBRANE

ENDOTHELIUM

BOWMAN'S MEMBRANE

TEARS

AQUEOUS

STROMA

The Drainage Angle (Figure 2.9)

Aqueous humour is a watery fluid which fills the anterior and posterior chambers. It brings nutrients to the cornea and lens and removes waste products from them. This is necessary because the cornea and lens are avascular. (Blood vessels would impair their transparency.)

Aqueous is formed continuously by the ciliary body and secreted into the posterior chamber (the tiny space between the iris and lens). It passes through the pupil into the anterior chamber and then drains, through spaces in the trabecular meshwork, into Schlemm's canal. This is a circular channel which lies adjacent to the trabecular meshwork (Figure 2.10). It can be seen only with a gonioscope. From Schlemm's canal aqueous passes into the blood stream via special 'aqueous veins' which empty into the episcleral veins.

Normally aqueous secretion and outflow just balance one another so that the intraocular pressure is maintained at between 12mm Hg and 20mm Hg. If the outflow of aqueous is impaired for any reason, then the intraocular pressure will rise (see chapter 16).

Figure 2.9: The Drainage Angle

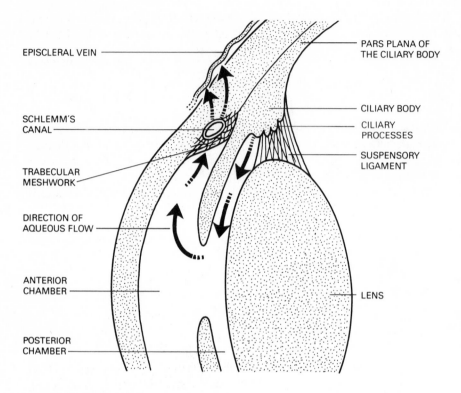

Figure 2.10: Schlemm's Canal

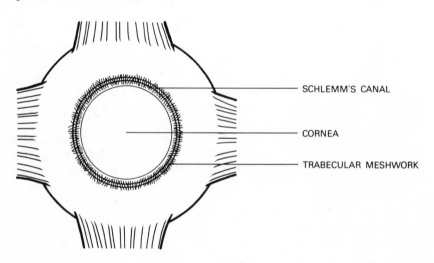

Uveal Tract

The uvea, or uveal tract, is the middle vascular and pigmented coat of the eye (Figure 2.7). The iris and ciliary body make up the anterior uvea. The choroid is also known as the posterior uvea.

Iris

The iris consists of an anterior layer of muscle and a posterior layer of black pigment. It contains blood vessels and nerves so that injury to it may cause bleeding and pain. The anterior layer also contains a variable amount of pigment which determines whether the iris appears blue or brown. There is a circular ring of muscle at the pupil margin, the sphincter pupillae. More peripherally, radially orientated muscle fibres form the dilator pupillae (Figure 2.11).

Figure 2.11: The Pupillary Muscles

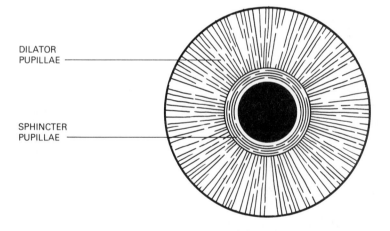

DILATOR
PUPILLAE

SPHINCTER
PUPILLAE

Pupil

The pupil is a hole in the iris. It normally appears black because no light is reflected back through it. Its size is determined by the opposing actions of the pupillary muscles. When the dilator contracts, the pupil enlarges (mydriasis); this may be due to stimulation by the sympathetic nervous system, via the ciliary nerves, or to circulating adrenaline. When the sphincter contracts the pupil constricts (miosis); this is due to stimulation by the parasympathetic nervous system via the oculomotor (third cranial) nerve.

The Light Reflex (Figure 2.12)

When light falls on the retina, impulses pass in special pupillary fibres to the third nerve nucleus in the brain stem. From here impulses pass back to the eye via the oculomotor nerve causing contraction of the sphincter muscle and miosis. In this way the amount of light entering the eye is automatically regulated by the pupil size.

Miosis also occurs when the eye accommodates for near vision (see below). In addition, the pupil size is altered by many drugs and disease states (see chapters 8 and 20). The pupils tend to become smaller with age (senile miosis).

Figure 2.12: The Light Reflex

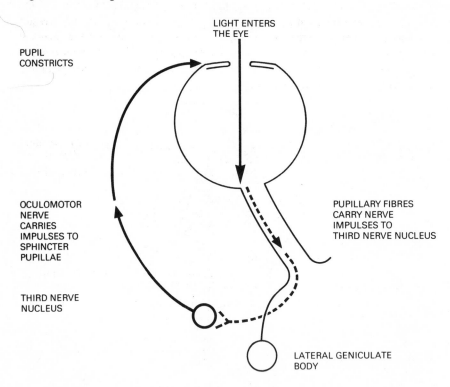

LIGHT ENTERS THE EYE

PUPIL CONSTRICTS

OCULOMOTOR NERVE CARRIES IMPULSES TO SPHINCTER PUPILLAE

PUPILLARY FIBRES CARRY NERVE IMPULSES TO THIRD NERVE NUCLEUS

THIRD NERVE NUCLEUS

LATERAL GENICULATE BODY

Ciliary Body

The ciliary body lies circumferentially behind the root of the iris. Its anterior part is made up of the ciliary muscle and about 70 ciliary processes (Figure 2.9). To these processes are attached the zonular fibres from which the lens is suspended. Contraction of the circular ciliary muscle causes slackening of the zonular fibres so that the tension in the lens capsule is reduced and the lens is able to take up its more spherical form. This is the means by which the focusing of the lens is increased (accommodation). Contraction of the ciliary muscle also opens up the gaps in the trabecular meshwork. (This is the reason for prescribing pilocarpine for patients with open angle glaucoma.) The ciliary processes secrete aqueous into the posterior chamber. The posterior part of the ciliary body is known as the pars plana. Instruments may be passed into the vitreous cavity via the pars plana so avoiding the retina.

Choroid (Figure 2.13)

The choroid consists mainly of blood vessels which bring nourishment to the outer half of the retina. It may be the source of copious bleeding either as a result of trauma or when an instrument is passed through it, as during the drainage of sub-retinal fluid at the time of retinal detachment surgery. Bruch's membrane is the membrane lying between the retina and the choroid to which the retinal pigment epithelial cells gain attachment.

Figure 2.13: Retina and Choroid

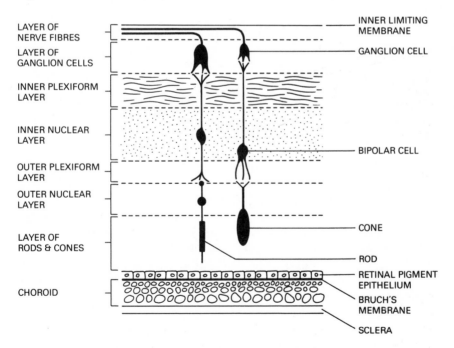

Lens (Figures 2.14 and 2.15)

The lens is made of clear fibres enclosed by an elastic capsule. New fibres are added throughout life. The younger fibres form the outer cortex. The older fibres are pushed inwards to form the central nucleus.

The lens is attached to the zonule or suspensory ligament. When the eye is at rest there is enough tension in the zonule to pull the lens into a flattened disc which allows parallel rays of light from distant objects to be brought to a focus on the retina. When the ciliary muscle contracts, it acts like a purse string pulling the ciliary body into a smaller circle. This reduces the tension in the zonule and causes the lens to assume a more spherical shape so allowing the diverging rays from near objects to be brought to a focus on the retina. This is the process of accommodation for near vision (see chapter 3).

Figure 2.14: The Lens and Suspensory Ligament

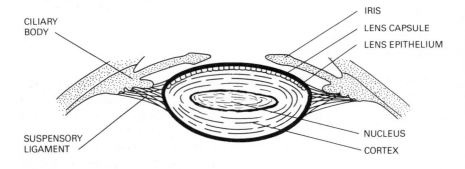

Vitreous

The vitreous is a colourless jelly that fills the vitreous cavity which lies behind the lens. It is attached to the optic disc, the ora serrata and, in young people, to the back of the lens. (Thus removing the lens 'in toto', as in the intracapsular technique, is not attempted in young people. Traction on the lens would inevitably cause loss of vitreous with the likelihood of major complications developing.) The vitreous is avascular (except before birth) and contains few cells. Blood and inflammatory products are cleared very slowly from it. The vitreous gel does not regenerate; if lost during an operation or at the time of injury it is replaced by aqueous.

Figure 2.15: The Lens a. At Rest b. in Accommodation

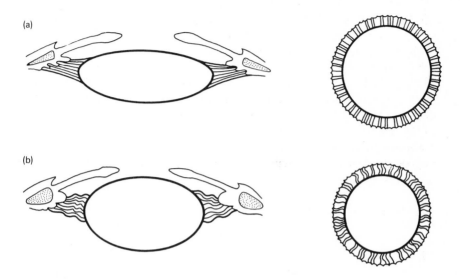

Retina (Figure 2.13)

The retina is the innermost and the light sensitive layer of the eye. It has a complex structure with many different types of cells and fibres within it. The rods and cones are sensitive to the light which reaches them. They contain various visual pigments. They pass impulses to the bipolar cells which, in turn, send impulses to the ganglion cells, whose fibres run from the surface of the retina to form the optic nerve. All these structures are transparent, as light must pass through them in order to reach the photoreceptors (rods and cones). The retinal pigment epithelium is opaque and absorbs the light which reaches it.

The retina becomes thinner towards the periphery, where it comes to an end as the ora serrata. The macula (Figure 2.16) is a thicker area surrounding the central foveal pit. The fovea has no ganglion cells, bipolar cells or rods — but only cones. It is especially adapted for good visual acuity in daylight. The rest of the retina contains a mixture of rods and cones. The more peripheral part of the retina is used for the detection of movement and for night vision. The inner half of the retina is supplied by the retinal circulation. The outer half is supplied from the choroidal circulation via the retinal pigment epithelium.

Figure 2.16: The Macula and Optic Nerve Head

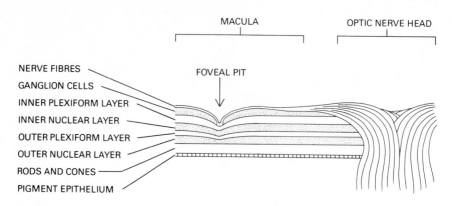

Visual Acuity

The visual acuity is usually measured by testing the patient's ability to read a Snellen chart six metres away from him (Figure 2.17) (see chapter 5). A vision of 6/6 is considered normal. The near visual acuity is also important; it is measured by testing the patient's ability to read standardised test types (Figure 2.18). A vision of N.5 is considered normal.

Normal vision is only achieved when a focused image of the test type falls on the normal fovea (see chapter 3). If another part of the retina is used, because the fovea is diseased (for example in senile macular degeneration — see chapter 19), then the visual acuity will probably be less than 6/60. Good lighting is also essential for good visibility (see below).

Visual Field

The normal visual field is the area within which a target can be seen whilst the eye is viewing an object straight ahead (Figure 2.19). The normal field extends far out temporally but it is limited above by the brow, below by the cheek and medially by the nose. The extent of the peripheral field may be assessed by moving an object, such as a white-headed hat pin, centrally from the periphery and noting the point at which it is first seen. A permanent record (albeit on a flat piece of paper) may be made with a perimeter (Figure 2.20).

Defects in the visual field are called scotomata. They may be due to lesions of the retina, or, alternatively, the optic pathways. Scotomata appear in the quadrant of the visual field opposite to that of the causative lesion in the retina. Hence, the optic disc, which lies nasal to the macula, causes a blind spot which is in the

Figure 2.17: Snellen Chart

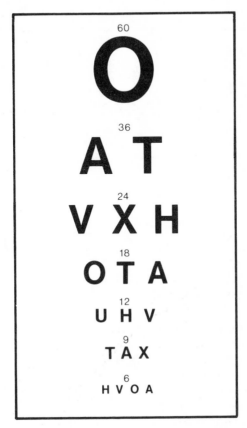

temporal half of the visual field. Scotomata may be plotted with various types of field testing apparatus (for example, Bjerrum's screen, Friedmann Visual Field Analyser, Goldmann Perimeter).

Colour Vision

The colours of the rainbow and of everyday objects can be seen whenever there is enough light for the cones to function. There are thought to be three types of cone, containing different pigments, which detect red, green and blue, the primary colours of light.

There are several types of colour blindness. The most common is an inability to distinguish between red and green. It may be detected using the Ishihara Colour Test Plates. These consist of cards with numerous coloured dots on them. A normal individual sees a number amongst the dots; but someone who is colour blind cannot discern the numbers.

Figure 2.18: Standardised Test Types

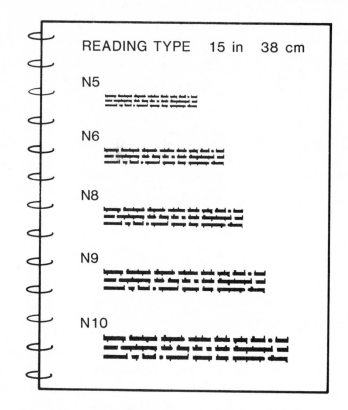

Figure 2.19: The Visual Field of the Right Eye

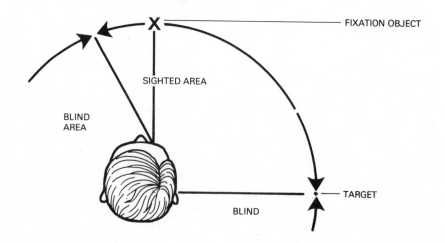

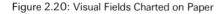

Figure 2.20: Visual Fields Charted on Paper

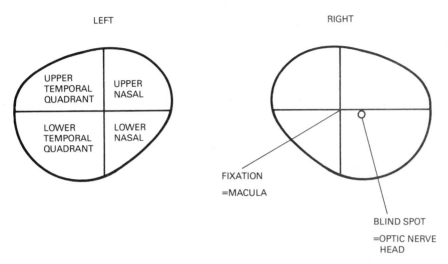

Dark-Light Adaptation

On first entering a darkened room, even a normal person's vision is quite poor. However, his vision gradually improves over about half an hour. During this time the visual pigments begin to regenerate and make the photoreceptors more sensitive to light. Rods function better than cones in the dark. They are more sensitive to light than cones but they do not permit colour vision or a good visual acuity.

On returning to a lighted room, the normal person's vision improves rapidly. The visual pigments bleach and become less sensitive to light. The cones begin to function better so that colour appreciation and good visual acuity return.

The adjustment to different levels of illumination is assisted by the pupillary responses (see above).

The Electroretinogram

The front of the eye has a positive electrical charge relative to the back of the eye. This is due to electrical activity in the retina. This activity ceases when the retina is severely damaged by injury or disease (for example in retinitis pigmentosa). The electro-retinogram and electro-oculogram measure the amount of electrical activity in the retina as a whole. The visual evoked response is a measure of electrical activity at the macula alone. These tests are usually only available in particularly well equipped departments. Very young children may need a general anaesthetic before these tests can be carried out.

Optic Nerve (Figure 2.7)

The optic nerve carries nerve fibres from the retina to the brain. The optic disc, or papilla, is the area where the nerve fibres leave the retina to pierce the sclera and form the optic nerve. There are no photoreceptors on the disc, so accounting for the blind spot in the visual field.

The optic nerve is encased by both pia-arachnoid and dura mater in just the same way as the brain is. The central retinal artery pierces the optic nerve about 1 cm behind the globe to reach the inside of the eye. The central retinal vein leaves by the same route.

Visual Pathway (Figure 2.21)

The optic nerves join at the optic chiasm. From the chiasm fibres run in the optic tracts to the lateral geniculate bodies. From there new fibres run in the optic radiations to the occipital cortices.

Fibres from the nasal halves of the retinae cross at the chiasm but fibres from the temporal retinae do not cross. This means that fibres from the left halves of the two retinae run to the left side of the brain. Hence the left side of the brain is concerned with vision in the right half of the visual field, just as the left side of the brain controls the right arm and leg. (A patient with a right-sided stroke may well have, in addition, a right homonymous hemianopia.)

Occipital Cortex (Figure 2.22)

When impulses from the eyes reach the brain, the retinal images can finally be appreciated by the conscious person. The tip of the occipital lobe receives impulses from the macula; the remaining part of the lobe receives impulses from the peripheral retina

Blood Supply of the Visual Pathways

The visual pathways are supplied by arteries derived from the internal carotid and basilar arteries which join to form the circle of Willis. Aneurysms on the cir-

Figure 2.21: The Visual Pathways

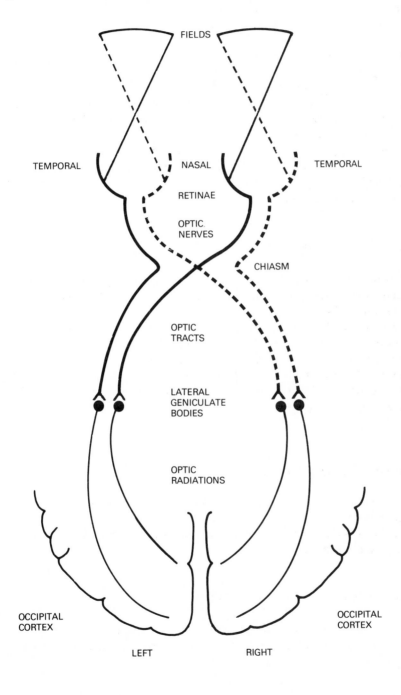

Figure 2.22: The Visual Cortex

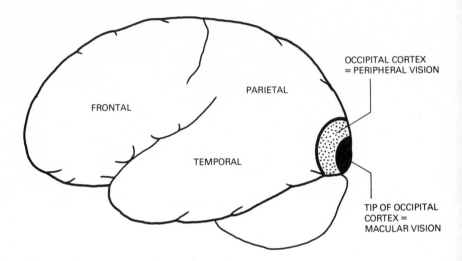

cle of Willis or occlusion of its branches may cause visual problems (see chapter 20).

The ophthalmic artery and its branches supply all the structures in the orbit. The central retinal artery pierces the optic nerve and passes through it. It emerges at the optic disc where it divides into branches and supplies the inner layers of the retina (Figure 2.23).

The blood supply to the optic nerve is from the posterior ciliary arteries. The choroid and outer part of the retina receive blood from the short ciliary arteries.

Cranial Nerves (Table 2.1)

There are twelve pairs of cranial nerves which carry nerve fibres to and from the brain.

Autonomic Nervous System

Some bodily functions — for example, secretions from glands and contractions of certain muscles — are not under conscious control but are regulated by the involuntary or autonomic nervous system. This is divided into two groups of nerves. Sympathetic nerves put the body in readiness for 'fright', 'flight' and 'fight'. Parasympathetic nerves control more relaxed functions such as digestion.

Figure 2.23: Blood Supply of the Visual Pathways

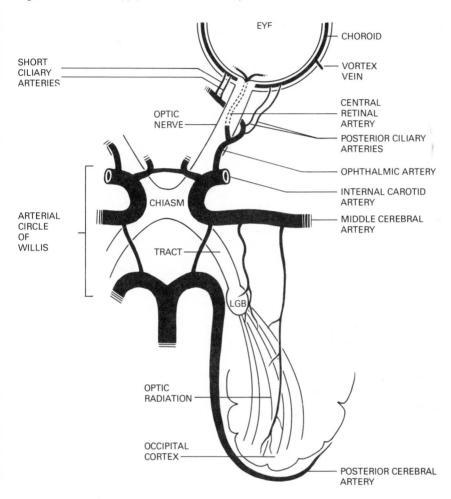

Transmitter Substances

These are chemicals released when a nerve impulse reaches the nerve ending. They act on the muscle or gland supplied by the nerve (Figure 2.24).

Autonomic Nerves and the Eye

Sympathetic nerves act on Müller's muscle which lifts the upper lid and also on the dilator pupillae. Thus in a 'fright', 'flight' or 'fight' situation, the eyes are wide open and the pupils dilated.

Table 2.1: The Cranial Nerves

I	Olfactory Nerve	— Carries fibres from the nasal mucosa.
II	Optic Nerve	— Carries visual fibres from the retina.
III	Oculomotor nerve	— Carries motor fibres to all the extraocular muscles except the superior oblique and the lateral rectus. The third cranial nerve also supplies the levator muscle. Also carries parasympathetic fibres to the pupil and the ciliary muscle.
IV	Trochlear Nerve	— Carries motor fibres to the superior oblique muscle.
V	Trigeminal Nerve	— Divides into three branches.
V^1	Ophthalmic Branch	— Carries sensory fibres from the forehead and the eye.
V^2	Maxillary Branch	— Carries sensory fibres from the cheek.
V^3	Mandibular Branch	— Carries sensory fibres from the lower lip and the teeth.
VI	Abducent Nerve	— Carries motor fibres to the lateral rectus muscle.
VII	Facial Nerve	— Carries motor fibres to the muscles of the face and eyelids. (Orbicularis oculi muscle only).
		— Often damaged during operations for the removal of an acoustic neuroma or in Bell's palsy.
		— Facial nerve block is used in local anaesthesia for cataract extraction (see chapter 8).
VIII	Acoustic (Vestibular Cochlear) Nerve	— Carries sensory fibres from the ear.
		— May develop a tumour (acoustic neuroma).
IX	Glossopharyngeal Nerve	
X	Vagus Nerve	
XI	Accessory Nerve	
XII	Hypoglossal Nerve	

Parasympathetic nerves act on the sphincter pupillae, ciliary muscle and lacrimal gland causing pupillary constriction, accommodation and secretion of tears.

Drugs

Some drugs act on the muscles and glands which are normally controlled by the autonomic nervous system. They may be actual transmitter substances or similar chemicals. Thus adrenaline and phenylephrine (which are similar to

Figure 2.24: The Autonomic Nervous System

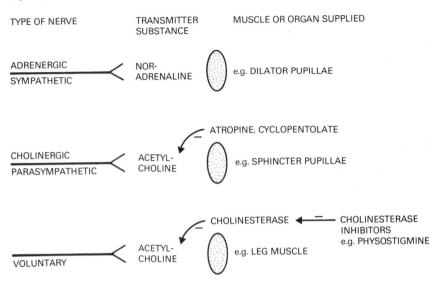

TYPE OF NERVE   TRANSMITTER   MUSCLE OR ORGAN SUPPLIED
SUBSTANCE

ADRENERGIC   NOR-ADRENALINE   e.g. DILATOR PUPILLAE
SYMPATHETIC

ATROPINE, CYCLOPENTOLATE

CHOLINERGIC   ACETYL-CHOLINE   e.g. SPHINCTER PUPILLAE
PARASYMPATHETIC

CHOLINESTERASE ← CHOLINESTERASE INHIBITORS e.g. PHYSOSTIGMINE

ACETYL-CHOLINE   e.g. LEG MUSCLE
VOLUNTARY

noradrenaline) dilate the pupil. They are called adrenergic or sympathomimetic drugs. Acetylcholine (Miochol) and similar drugs, for example, pilocarpine, cause miosis and increased accommodation. They are cholinergic or parasympathomimetic drugs.

Some drugs antagonise the action of transmitter substances. For instance, atropine dilates the pupil and paralyses accommodation because it antagonises the effect of acetylcholine at parasympathetic nerve endings. It is an anticholinergic drug.

Another important group of drugs is the cholinesterase inhibitors. Normally the acetylcholine released from voluntary and parasympathetic nerves is rapidly destroyed by the enzyme cholinesterase, so that each package of acetylcholine released by a nerve impulse has only a short lasting effect. Cholinesterase inhibitors such as physostigmine, neostigmine and phospholine iodine prevent the action of cholinesterase, so that each package of acetylcholine remains at the nerve ending much longer. Thus physostigmine (Eserine) drops cause a long lasting miosis.

Extraocular Muscles (Figures 2.25, 2.26 and 2.27)

The four rectus muscles are inserted in front of the equator and the two obliques behind it. The lateral rectus is supplied by the abducent nerve and the superior oblique by the trochlear nerve. The other muscles are supplied by the oculomotor nerve. The extraocular muscles cause not only horizontal and verti-

Figure 2.25: The Extra-ocular Muscles (Left Eye)

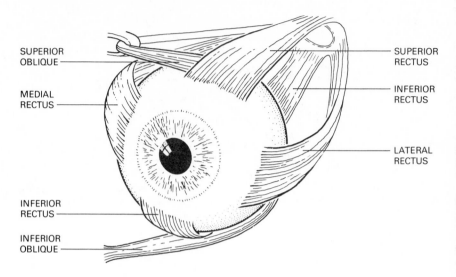

Figure 2.26: Actions of the Extra-ocular Muscles (Left Eye)

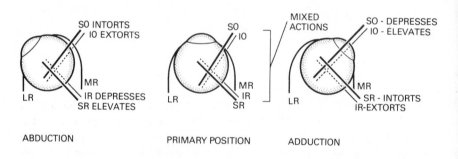

cal movements but also clockwise and anticlockwise rotations of the globe (torsions).

The lateral rectus muscle abducts the eye and turns the cornea outwards. The medial rectus adducts the eye and turns the cornea inwards. The actions of the other muscles depend upon the position of the eye. When the eye is abducted the superior rectus elevates the cornea and the inferior rectus depresses it; in this position the superior oblique intorts the eye and the inferior oblique extorts it (that is, the 12 o'clock point on the cornea moves nasally and temporally respectively).

When the eye is adducted the inferior oblique elevates the cornea and the superior oblique depresses it; in this position the superior rectus intorts the eye

Figure 2.27: Eye Movements (Left Eye)

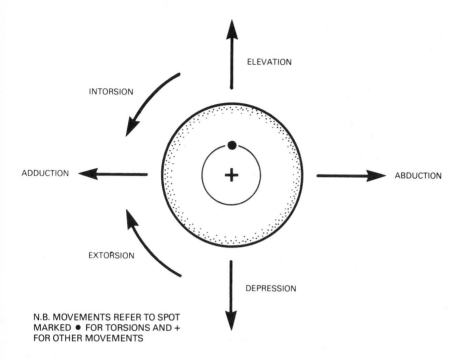

ELEVATION

INTORSION

ADDUCTION

ABDUCTION

EXTORSION

DEPRESSION

N.B. MOVEMENTS REFER TO SPOT
MARKED ● FOR TORSIONS AND +
FOR OTHER MOVEMENTS

and the inferior rectus extorts it.

When the eye is looking straight ahead (the primary position) elevation is caused by both the superior rectus and the inferior oblique and depression is due to both the inferior rectus and the superior oblique. Intorsion is brought about by the superior rectus and the superior oblique and extorsion by the inferior rectus and the inferior oblique.

Control of Eye Movements

Some eye movements are voluntary; they are controlled by the cerebral cortex. Others are involuntary and are controlled by the brain stem and by the labyrinth of the inner ear. For example, turning the eyes to look at the clock is a voluntary movement but the rapid eye movements that take place as one looks out of a window of a moving train are involuntary (opto-kinetic nystagmus, see chapter 20).

Normally the eyes move as a pair. For instance, on looking to the left, the left lateral rectus and right medial rectus receive an equal number of nerve impulses so that both eyes move in the same direction by the same amount. Even if the left lateral rectus is paralysed, this still applies, with the result that the right eye is moved inwards much more than the left eye is moved outwards, so that double vision results (see chapter 21).

3 OPTICS

We normally see whenever light enters our eyes. For clear vision the rays of light must be bent so that they meet at a point, or focus, on the retina (Figure 3.1). This bending of light is called *refraction*. It takes place at the front of the cornea and at the lens.

Figure 3.1: Emmetropia — Focusing on a Distant Object

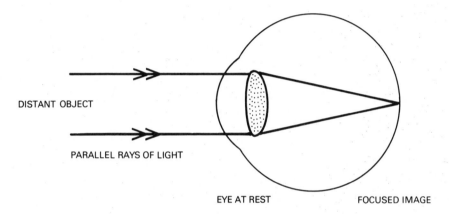

DISTANT OBJECT

PARALLEL RAYS OF LIGHT

EYE AT REST   FOCUSED IMAGE

Figure 3.2: Emmetropia — Focusing on a Near Object

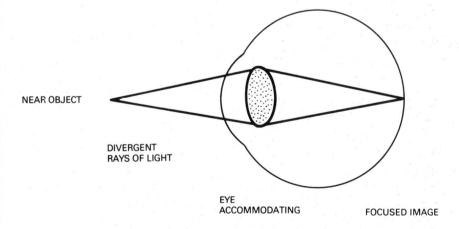

NEAR OBJECT

DIVERGENT
RAYS OF LIGHT

EYE
ACCOMMODATING   FOCUSED IMAGE

Emmetropia — Normal Refraction

Distant objects can be seen when the normal eye is at rest (that is, not accommodating). This is because light from distant objects travels in parallel lines and the refraction of the normal eyes is so arranged that parallel rays come to a focus on the retina. Near objects can only be seen clearly if the eye is accommodating when the lens becomes fatter or more convex (see chapter 2). This is because light from near objects spreads out or diverges as it approaches the eye and so needs to undergo more refraction for it to be focused on the retina (Figure 3.2).

Refractive Errors

These are not diseases but simply variations in the shape of the eye which prevent a clear retinal image being formed. They include myopia, hypermetropia, and astigmatism. Presbyopia refers to the progressive loss of the power of accommodation with increasing age. It is a normal phenomenon.

Myopia — Shortsightedness

The myopic eye is effectively too long. Light from a distant object comes to a focus in front of the retina. By the time the light reaches the retina it is diverging so that the retinal image is blurred (Figure 3.3).

Near objects can be seen clearly provided that the eye does not accommodate (Figure 3.4). A myope is said to be short-sighted because he can see things close to, although he cannot see distant objects clearly.

Myopia is corrected by wearing spectacles with concave lenses. These make parallel rays of light divergent as they enter the eye so that they appear to be coming from a near object and can be focused on the retina (Figure 3.5).

Eyes which are highly myopic (over six dioptres) often have abnormalities of the retina which predispose to macular degeneration and to retinal detachment. Even in the absence of these complications, spectacles may not give perfect vision in these cases.

Hypermetropia — Longsightedness

The hypermetropic eye is in effect too short. Light from a distant object comes to a focus behind the retina. However, if the eye accommodates, light can be focused and distant objects can be seen clearly. (Figure 3.6). Even more accommodation will be needed for near objects to be seen clearly. Young people may be able to produce this extra accommodation, but they often find that close work is uncomfortable. A squint may also develop (see chapter 21).

Figure 3.3: Myopia — Viewing a Distant Object

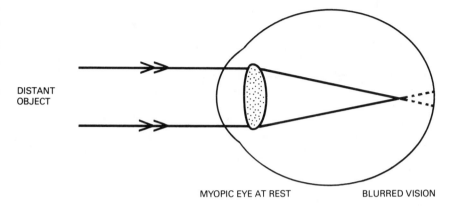

DISTANT
OBJECT

MYOPIC EYE AT REST   BLURRED VISION

Figure 3.4: Myopia — Viewing a Near Object

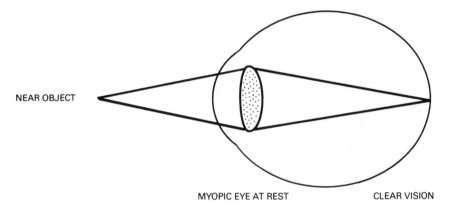

NEAR OBJECT

MYOPIC EYE AT REST   CLEAR VISION

Figure 3.5: Correction of Myopia

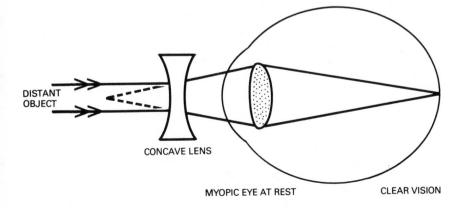

DISTANT
OBJECT

CONCAVE LENS

MYOPIC EYE AT REST   CLEAR VISION

Figure 3.6: Hypermetropia

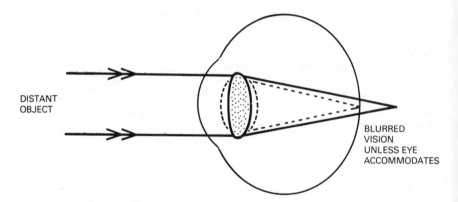

DISTANT
OBJECT

BLURRED
VISION
UNLESS EYE
ACCOMMODATES

Figure 3.7: Correction of Hypermetropia

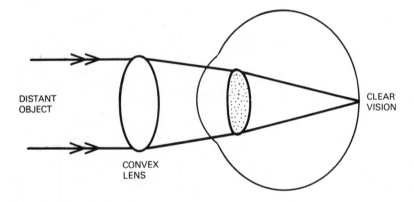

DISTANT
OBJECT

CLEAR
VISION

CONVEX
LENS

Older people are unable to produce the extra accommodation and so complain of blurred vision, at first for near objects and later for distant objects.

Hypermetropia is corrected by wearing spectacles with convex lenses. These converge parallel light rays before they enter the eye so that they can be focused on the retina without accommodation (Figure 3.7).

Astigmatism

The cornea of the normal eye is perfectly spherical, like the back of a ladle. In contrast, the astigmatic eye has a cornea which is not perfectly spherical. Instead it is curved like the back of a spoon. Some rays of light are bent more than others so that one meridian is in focus but the opposite one is blurred (Figure 3.8). Astigmatism is corrected by wearing cylindrical lenses. They are curved in one direction (or axis) only (Figure 3.9).

Figure 3.8: Retinal Image in Astigmatism

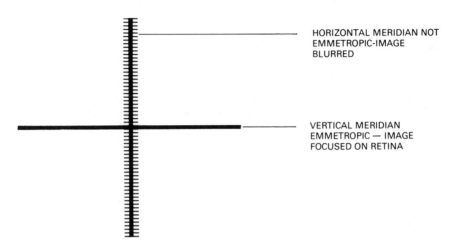

HORIZONTAL MERIDIAN NOT
EMMETROPIC-IMAGE
BLURRED

VERTICAL MERIDIAN
EMMETROPIC — IMAGE
FOCUSED ON RETINA

Figure 3.9: Cylinders

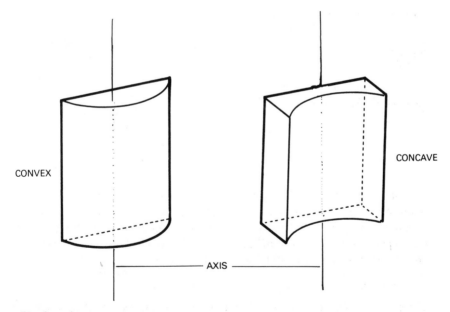

CONVEX

CONCAVE

AXIS

Presbyopia

With age, the lens becomes relatively stiff and inelastic. When the ciliary muscle contracts the old lens does not become as convex as a young lens. This means that accommodation for near vision becomes defective. The patient complains that he cannot read and he pushes the book well away from his eyes.

Presbyopia is corrected by wearing convex lenses for any activity that normally requires accommodation, for example, reading and sewing.

Spectacles

The strength of a spectacle lens is measured in dioptres. Convex spherical lenses are known as plus (+) spheres and concave spherical lenses as minus (−) spheres. Cylinders may be either convex or concave. A lens which has its principle focus at one metre distance is known as a 1.00 dioptre (1.00 D) lens. A lens twice this strength is a 2.00 D lens (Figure 3.10). The strength and type of lenses required may be measured in several ways.

Figure 3.10: The Power of a Spectacle Lens

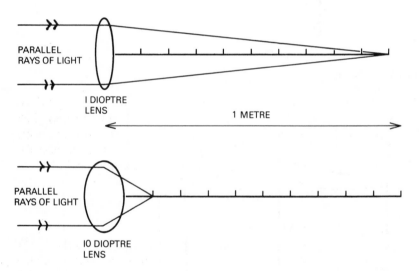

In retinoscopy the light from a retinoscope is shone into the patient's eye. The trained observer can judge from the light reflex seen in the pupil what strength of spectacle lens is required. This test does not require much co-operation from the patient and is thus known as an objective test. It is particularly suitable for children and illiterates. It may be carried out under general anaesthesia. It is often less accurate than subjective methods which involve the patient commenting upon the clarity of the symbols on the test chart. The lenses in a spectacle trial frame are altered until the best vision is obtained by a system of trial and error. Ideally, retinoscopy is performed first and then the findings checked subjectively.

A presbyopic patient who requires different lenses for distance and near vision

will require two pairs of spectacles, bifocals or a multifocal lens
(Figure 3.11).

Figure 3.11: Bifocals

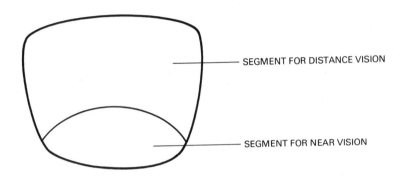

SEGMENT FOR DISTANCE VISION

SEGMENT FOR NEAR VISION

Contact Lenses

These are lenses worn on the tear film between the cornea and the eyelids.
Because contact lenses are closer to the refracting surfaces of the eye, they often
neutralise refractive errors better than spectacles. Their front surface is always
spherical so that low degrees of astigmatism are corrected without the need for
cylinders in the lenses. They have many advantages over spectacles but unlike
spectacles they carry certain risks to the eye.

Contact lenses are made of three types of material, as follows.

a.   Hard (Polymethylmethacrylate)

These are impermeable to gases or liquids. They may be corneal, scleral or apex
fitting (Figure 3.12). Because oxygen from the atmosphere can only reach the
tear film around the edge of the lens (or through fenestration holes) there is a risk
of corneal anoxia. Anoxia leads to corneal oedema which often causes discomfort and blurred vision and may cause the patient to see 'haloes' around lights.
Eventually corneal vascularisation may develop. Symptoms of anoxia are the
main cause of either intolerance to the lens or to a decreased wearing time.
Nevertheless, many individuals can wear such contact lenses happily all day
long.

Hard contact lenses give a good visual acuity. There is little risk of infection
provided that the patient takes reasonable hygienic precautions.

These lenses do not scratch or break easily (although corneals are easily lost),
so that one lens may last many years. Yearly checks are adequate once a patient
is fully adapted to the lens. Adaptation to hard lenses may take a month or so,
during which the wearing time should be increased slowly from two to three

Figure 3.12: Contact Lenses

(a) Corneal Contact Lens — Hard or Gas Permeable

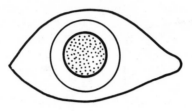

(b) Scleral (Haptic) Contact Lens — Hard or Gas Permeable

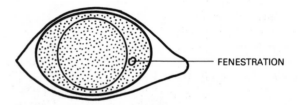

FENESTRATION

(c) Apex Fitting Contact Lens — Hard, Gas Permeable or Soft

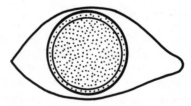

hours to eventually all day wear. They should not be worn during sleep. A major symptom of 'overwearing', due either to sleeping with the lenses in place or to a too rapid increase in wearing time, is pain due to corneal abrasions. The pain is often first experienced at night.

b. Soft (Hydrophilic)

These lenses are permeable to gases and liquids and have a high water content. Oxygen exchange is better than with hard lenses, so that corneal anoxia is unlikely. Adaptation is quicker and wearing times are longer. They may absorb and retain bacteria and chemicals (from cleaning solutions and drops) so that conjunctivitis and corneal infections are potential complications. Lipids and proteins from the tear film may become deposited on the lens and cause decreased vision and discomfort. Initially these deposits may be removed by either cleaning or boiling but eventually a new lens is required.

Fluorescein ruins soft lenses. It should never be used while a soft lens is on the eye. Following any examination in which fluorescein is used, the dye should be thoroughly washed out from the conjunctival sac before the lens is re-inserted.

Soft lenses are easily torn or otherwise damaged. They rarely last more than two years, so wearing soft contact lenses is expensive.

Soft lenses are floppy and mould somewhat to the surface of the eye. This makes them comfortable to wear but also difficult to insert and to handle. Elderly patients may find it impossible to cope with their daily removal and insertion so extended wear lenses may be preferable. These latter lenses have an even higher water content and may be worn continuously for three months. The risk of infection and deposit formation is high and this type of lens should be checked weekly at first and at least three monthly thereafter.

Soft lenses may not give such good vision as hard lenses, particularly when there is much corneal astigmatism, as in keratoconus.

c. Gas Permeable

These lenses are permeable to gases but not to liquids. They are intermediate between hard and soft contact lenses in cost, comfort and safety. They give a good visual acuity and are better tolerated than hard lenses because of their superior oxygen exchange. They are fitted and cleaned in the same way as hard lenses but deposits may form as in the case of soft lenses and they may require special treatment to clean them.

d. Tinted, Printed and Painted

These lenses may be used to hide an abnormal eye (e.g., one with an opaque cornea or lens) or to reduce photophobia when the iris is either translucent or absent.

Indications for Fitting a Contact Lens

a. *Cosmetic.* Even when their vision with spectacles is good many patients prefer their appearance when they wear contact lenses. This is particularly understandable when they need to wear thick spectacle lenses.

b.   Occupational. Contact lenses may be safer than glass spectacle lenses for ball games, and they are less prone to misting up in icy conditions, so that they suit skiers. Only hard scleral lenses are suitable for swimming. Corneals are displaced by water and soft lenses are spoilt by both chlorinated and salt water.

c.   Optical. Contact lenses give better vision than spectacles in high refractive errors and in keratoconus because the optical aberrations are less marked so that there is less distortion of the retinal image. These lenses also give a wider field of vision. When the refraction of the two eyes is very different (e.g., in unilateral aphakia, see chapter 17), contact lenses will allow the patient to achieve binocular vision whereas spectacle lenses cause diplopia.

d.   Therapeutic. Hard or soft ('bandage') scleral lenses provide a smooth surface for the lids to move over and they make patients more comfortable when they suffer from conditions such as bullous keratopathy, in which the corneal surface is irregular (chapter 13).

Contra-indications to Fitting a Contact Lens

Dryness of the eyes may preclude a patient wearing a contact lens. An adequate flow of tears is usually necessary for adequate oxygen exchange and hence comfort, and also for hydration of soft lenses. Patients with chronic blepharitis, hayfever or very sensitive eyes are unsuitable for contact lens wear.

Cleaning and Storage

A contact lens should be cleaned after removal from the eye. Different cleaning solutions are required for hard and soft lenses. Lenses are stored in special cases with separate compartments for right and left lenses. The case is filled with an antiseptic soaking solution which should be changed daily. Before the lens is inserted into the eye, the soaking solution should be rinsed off, and a wetting solution applied to both surfaces of the lens. The wetting solution decreases the discomfort of wearing the lens. In the case of soft and gas permeable lenses it may be necessary to remove protein deposits either with a special solution, or by boiling, at intervals.

Soft lenses may acquire a build-up of preservatives from either cleaning or soaking solutions. This may cause a chemical conjunctivitis with progressive intolerance to wearing the lens. Successful soft lens wear may be re-established if a patient cleans the lens by boiling it daily, in a special electrical lens boiler, and by using saline which is free of any preservative.

Removal and Insertion

This is best carried out with a patient sitting at a table which is covered with a white cloth so that a dropped lens can be located. (Contact lenses are slightly tinted.) Any corrective spectacles should be close to hand in case the lens is dropped. A mirror is also helpful. The cornea should be kept centrally placed by the patient gazing straight ahead.

To insert the lens the eyelids are held widely apart by placing the index and middle fingers of the left hand on the margins of the upper and lower lids respectively, while the wetted lens is balanced on the forefinger of the right hand and steadily brought towards the eye. Once the lens is in place on the cornea, first the upper lid and then the lower lid is released.

Some patients remove corneal lenses easily by first separating the lids widely, and then placing a forefinger on the globe at the outer canthus and, at the same time, gradually drawing the lids outwards. The upper lid breaks the surface tension of the tear film and dislodges the lens. Other patients remove corneal lenses by placing the index and middle fingers of the left hand on the upper lid margin and the right forefinger on the lower lid margin. The lids are pulled apart and then pushed back against the globe, then the upper lid is gradually pushed down to dislodge the upper edge of the lens. A nurse or doctor may remove a lens for the patient in the same way.

Soft lenses may be removed by initially holding the lid margins widely apart and then displacing the lens with a finger placed on the sclera. The lens may then be pinched off between thumb and forefinger. Rubber suckers may be used for both insertion and removal of a lens and they are particularly useful when a lens has slipped off the cornea onto the sclera.

When lenses are worn on both eyes, the right lens is usually marked with a dot or 'R' to distinguish it from the unmarked left lens.

Prisms

A prism is a wedged-shaped lens which bends light towards its base (Figure 3.13). This makes an object viewed through the prism appear nearer to the apex of the prism than it really is (Figure 3.14).

Figure 3.13: Prism

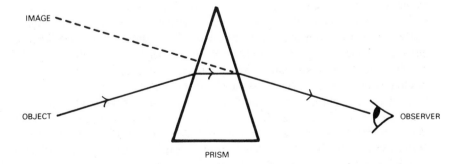

Figure 3.14: Prism

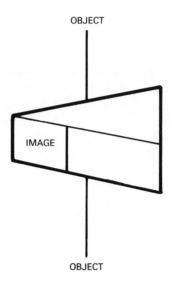

Prisms are used both in the diagnosis and treatment of patients with squints.

Low Vision Aids

These include magnifying glasses and 'telescopic' spectacles. They simply enlarge the retinal image, which often enables patients with a whole range of ocular disorders to see better. Those with macular degeneration and some forms of optic atrophy benefit particularly from their use. Unfortunately, the high magnification necessary means that the field of view is small. Thus a distance telescope is more suitable for viewing a stationary television screen than for watching a tennis match in the flesh. Similarly, for reading, only a few words can be seen in focus at any one time and scanning a page is impossible. The high magnification is also associated with a poor range of focus, so that the magnifier has to be held at just the right distance from the page for the print to remain in focus. Even a slight movement of either the magnifier or the reading material leads to blurring of the image. Many elderly people, with shaky, arthritic hands, find such accurate adjustments impossible. 'Stand' magnifiers, which have legs, so that the lens may be held fixed over a book or a newspaper placed on the table, may help to overcome these disadvantages.

4 HISTORY TAKING

Taking an accurate history is the first step towards making the correct diagnosis. Allowing the patient to tell his own story will usually provide much of the information necessary to come to the diagnosis. Later, relevant questions should be asked in order to complete the clinical picture. Some common eye symptoms are discussed below.

Pain

This ranges from mild discomfort, soreness or grittiness to severe aching which disturbs sleep. Conditions affecting the back of the eye are usually painless.

Photophobia

This is increased sensitivity to light. It may amount to actual pain.

Watering

This may be due to either obstruction of the tear passages or a painful eye condition (see chapter 11).

Discharge

Some conjunctival conditions cause a discharge of pus or mucus. Patients may describe this as 'stickiness', 'sleep' or 'matter' (see chapter 12).

Blurred Vision

Usually this complaint is accompanied by a measurable drop in visual acuity for near or distance (see chapter 5). Occasionally, it is an inaccurate description of field loss, diplopia or some other visual disturbance. The duration of blurred vision is important, as recent, sudden visual loss requires urgent investigation.

Field Loss

Some observant patients notice field loss in either one or both eyes. However, others simply complain that they bump into things or that they miss part of a line of print.

Diplopia (Double Vision)

This means that two images are seen instead of one. It may be constant or intermittent. It may be present for both near and distant vision — or either alone. It may be binocular, i.e., only present when both eyes are open, or monocular, namely still present when one eye is closed. Severe diplopia of recent onset may cause dizziness or even nausea.

Haloes

The patient complains that lights (e.g., from car headlights) are surrounded by coloured circles of light, like rainbows. They may be due to corneal oedema, which occurs in acute glaucoma.

Flashes and Floaters

A complaint of bright flashes of light often denotes tearing of the retina (see chapter 19). Floaters are black spots which move with eye movements; they are caused by opacities in the vitreous (see chapter 18). A new and prominent floater may be due to either a vitreous detachment or bleeding from the retina.

Other Types of Visual Disturbance

Migraine sufferers often experience coloured flashes of light, sometimes forming patterns, followed by the onset of field defects and a headache. Patients with macular disease may complain that things look smaller with the affected eye (micropsia) or that colours are altered. True hallucinations (seeing formed images or pictures) may occur in disorders of the temporal lobe of the brain.

Past Medical History

Serious medical disorders, accidents or operations should all be recorded. They may be the underlying cause of the eye problem (see chapter 22) or be relevant to the patient's fitness for general anaesthesia. It is also important to know what drugs the patient is taking (see chapter 8) and to record any allergies.

Family History

Many eye problems (e.g., glaucoma and squint) run in families, so that patients should be asked if relatives have had either eye disorders or eye operations.

Other Details

The patients' occupation, their social background, and their consumption of both tobacco and alcohol may be relevant to their problem. In the case of children, any medical problems arising during the mother's pregnancy or at the time of birth should be noted. A history of the baby needing oxygen should also be recorded.

5 EXAMINATION OF THE EYE

Many patients are afraid of having their eyes examined. Therefore, whenever possible, their fears should be allayed by careful explanation and sympathetic reassurance. It may be necessary to instil local anaesthetic drops before a painful eye can be fully examined. The visual acuities and the visual fields should be checked first, as other examination procedures (e.g., dilatation of the pupil and examinations involving placing instruments on the cornea), may cause blurring of the patient's vision.

Visual Acuity

The visual acuity of both eyes of every patient should be checked however trivial the problem may seem to be. Any distance glasses, even if they have been prescribed only for television or driving, should be worn for the test. If the glasses are not available, or if the vision is poor, the test can be carried out with a pin-hole in front of the eye. The vision will usually improve if a refractive error alone is present.

Each eye in turn should be completely covered with a card and the patient asked to read down an illuminated Snellen chart placed six metres away from him (see chapter 2). If the patient is unable to see the top letter at six metres, the test should be repeated at five metres. The best vision obtained is recorded as a fraction. The upper number (the numerator) indicates the distance, in metres, that the patient was from the chart. The lower number (denominator) denotes the line read by the patient. Each line is given a number (60, 36, 18, etc.) which indicates the distance, again in metres, at which someone with normal eyesight would be able to read that particular line. For instance, 6/12 indicates that, from a distance of six metres, the patient reads the line which would be read at 12 metres by someone with a normally seeing eye. If the patient is unable to see any letters, then their ability to count fingers (CF), or to see hand movements (HM) or merely to perceive light (PL) should be recorded.

Visual Field (see chapter 2)

Colour Vision (see chapter 2)

External Eye Examination

This is best carried out using a bright torch and a magnifying lens. A slit-lamp microscope is ideal, for this instrument combines a high-powered binocular microscope and an adjustable beam of light.

Eyelids

Abnormal signs include inflammatory changes, bruising, and various swellings. Watering, discharge or any excessive screwing up of the eyes (blepharospasm) should be noted. The lid margins should be examined for entropion, ectropion or trichiasis (see chapter 10).

Conjunctiva

Common abnormal signs are redness and conjunctival oedema (chemosis). The lower fornix may be inspected by pulling down the lower lid. The conjunctiva lining the upper lid may be seen only by everting the lid. To do this, the patient is asked to look downwards, whilst keeping the eyes open. Then the lashes of the upper lid are grasped between finger and thumb and the lid is 'flipped' over a glass rod which should be held gently along the middle of the upper lid as shown (Figure 5.1). It is necessary to carry out this manoeuvre in order to detect a subtarsal foreign body. Irrigation of the upper fornix may be helpful in removing multiple foreign bodies from this part of the conjunctival sac.

Figure 5.1: Eversion of Upper Lid

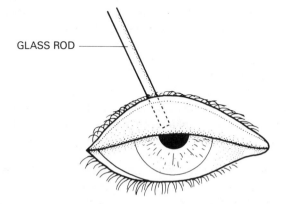

GLASS ROD

Cornea

This is normally clear and bright like a mirror. Abnormalities include any dullness, cloudiness or opacity (see chapter 13). Fluorescein drops should be instilled to show up ulcers and abrasions (see chapter 8).

Anterior Chamber

A fluid level due to either pus (hypopyon) or blood (hyphaema) is a serious abnormality (Figure 5.2). Blood cells and 'flare' (due to the aqueous having a high protein content) can only be detected by using high magnification (see chapter 15). Either shallowness or absence of the anterior chamber (a 'flat' AC) is best detected by looking at the eye from the side.

Figure 5.2: Fluid Level in the Anterior Chamber

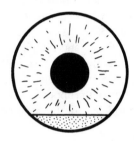

Pupil

A normal pupil is round, central and equal in size to that of the fellow eye. It should become smaller when a bright light falls upon the eye. Any abnormality of the pupils' reaction to light may denote a serious eye problem.

Internal Eye Examination

Examination of either the retina or the vitreous is usually performed by a member of the medical staff. A direct or indirect ophthalmoscope or a slit-lamp microscope (with a three-mirror contact lens or Hruby lens) may be used (Figure 5.3 to Figure 5.6).

The pupil should always be dilated with drops to allow a complete examination of the whole retina. However, an adequate view of the optic disc can often be obtained with the direct ophthalmoscope through a normal sized pupil. The indirect ophthalmoscope may be fitted with a mirror which enables two onlookers to observe the retina, although their view is not as good as that of the user of the ophthalmoscope.

Figure 5.3: Direct Ophthalmoscope

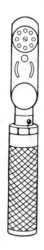

Intraocular Pressure

This is best checked using the Goldmann Applanation Tonometer (Figure 5.7) which fits on the slit-lamp. If the patient is confined to bed, then either the Perkins hand-held tonometer (Figure 5.8) or the Schiötz tonometer (Figure 5.9) may be used. A very abnormal pressure (either much too high or much too low) may be detected by 'digital tonometry'. The patient is asked to look downwards and the globe (covered by the upper lid) is lightly palpated between the two forefingers.

Gonioscopy (see chapter 16)

Other Investigations

Blood Pressure and Urine

These should both be checked on the patient's admission to hospital and also in the Out-Patient Department if an underlying medical disorder is suspected (see chapter 22).

Figure 5.4: Indirect Ophthalmoscopy

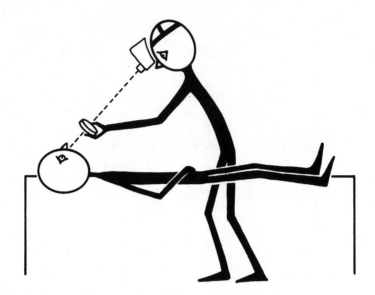

Figure 5.5: Slit-lamp Microscope and Hruby Lens

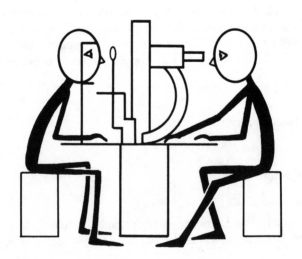

Figure 5.6: Three-mirror Contact Lens

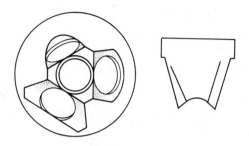

Figure 5.7: The Applanation Tonometer

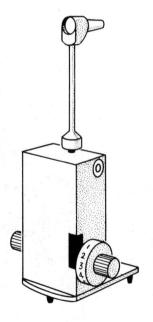

Figure 5.8: Perkins Tonometer

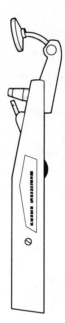

Figure 5.9: The Schiötz Tonometer

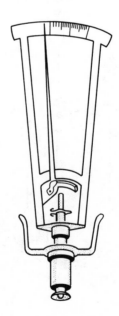

Full Blood Counts and ESR

These may be requested as part of the investigation of a patient with a vascular disorder or uveitis.

X-Rays, Tomograms, CT Scanning, Ultrasonography

These examinations may be necessary to investigate orbital disease, trauma, intraocular foreign bodies and neurological disorders (see chapters 9, 20 and 23).

Flourescein Angiography, Electrodiagnostic Tests, and Photography (see chapter 19)

Conjunctival and Corneal Swabs (see chapter 7)

6 THE OPHTHALMIC THEATRE, OUT-PATIENT DEPARTMENT AND CASUALTY

The ophthalmic theatre should have a quiet and peaceful atmosphere. Any unexpected noise and even the slightest movement, particularly of the operating table drapes, may create problems for the surgeon. Closed circuit television makes it possible for onlookers to watch operations without disturbing the operating team.

Eye operations are usually performed with the surgeon and assistant, and often the theatre sister, comfortably seated. The patient's head should lie just above the surgeon's lap. A microscope or magnifying glasses are frequently used. These restrict the surgeon's field of vision. Consequently, instruments should be put firmly into his hand so that he has no need to look away from the operating field. For retinal surgery, the indirect ophthalmoscope is used and the theatre will need to be 'blacked out' at times. Most eye surgeons wear gloves and these should be washed with sterile water to remove any starch powder.

Anaesthesia

Although most operations on adults can be performed under local anaesthesia (see chapter 8), many surgeons prefer the use of general anaesthesia. This may involve artificial ventilation. All wires and tubing should be kept clear of the operative field. The anaesthetist usually sits towards the patient's feet.

Checking the Eye

Once the patient is suitably anaesthetised, a further check is made as to which eye is to be operated upon. All concerned should check the hospital notes against the patient's identification tag and satisfy themselves which eye is due for surgery.

Preparation

Some surgeons prefer the patient's lashes to be cut before they embark upon intraocular surgery. This is usually carried out on the ward but occasionally it is done in theatre.

The lids of the eye in question, together with the adjacent parts of the surrounding cheek, nose and forehead, are gently wiped with a swab soaked in a

56

cleansing solution. The lid margins may have crusts on them and so harbour infective organisms. These parts of the lids should be carefully cleaned first. Subsequently, those areas of skin further away from the eye should be cleaned in a stepwise fashion. Skin preparation proceeds from the eye outwards.

Draping

The patient's head is immobilised in a circular head-rest or on a Ruben's pillow. The head is wrapped firmly in towels to which sutures can be clipped. The face and body are covered with drapes which incorporate a hole through which the eye is exposed.

Instruments

Ophthalmic instruments are delicate and they are easily damaged. They are usually kept in sets in metal boxes which have removable trays. This arrangement protects the instruments and facilitates their storage and sterilisation. Particularly fragile instruments are packed separately in either glass tubes or double paper wrappings. After use all instruments should be checked for perfect alignment — of teeth in the case of forceps, and blades in the case of scissors. Knives are tested for sharpness by lancing pieces of kid skin which are mounted taut on small drums. Scissors are checked by cutting strands of cotton wool.

Some larger items of equipment used in theatre include magnets, diathermy and cryotherapy machines, xenon arc photocoagulators and vitreous infusion suction cutting instruments.

Sterilisation

Dry Heat — Hot Air Oven

This is the method of choice for instruments made of carbon steel, which rusts in moist heat. The oven is kept at 160° for one hour (as shown by an automatic recording device), or 150° for one and a half hours. This latter method should be used for sterilising knives, for they are damaged at higher temperatures.

Proof of sterilisation by dry heat depends on using Browne's tubes in each cycle. These tubes contain a red liquid which becomes dark green after it has been subjected to the correct temperature for a requisite period. The temperature reached in the oven should be checked every three or four months by the use of thermocouples. This testing is carried out by the hospital engineer.

Moist Heat — Autoclave

This is the method of choice for sterilising gowns, drapes, metal bowls, rubber devices, cautery leads, airways and titanium instruments. Three minutes at 135°C and 30 lb/square inch steam pressure is sufficient. Items are wrapped in special paper which is impermeable to bacteria at relatively low temperatures. Sterilisation should be checked by placing a piece of heat-sensitive tape in the form of a cross, in the centre of a pack of towels before it is placed in the autoclave. The appropriate change in the colour of the tape after removal of the pack from the autoclave shows that the proper conditions for sterilisation were attained. This Bowie-Dick test should be carried out each day. The autoclave should be checked for any leak by the engineer at least once a week.

Chemical Methods

These include sterilisation with ethylene oxide, glutaraldehyde and for-maldehyde. These chemicals are used for sterilising pieces of equipment which are heat-sensitive, such as cryoprobes, lenses used for indirect ophthalmoscopy and anaesthetic tubing.

Proof of sterilisation depends upon bacteriological monitoring. Paper packets containing spores sprinkled on pieces of foil are included in each sterilisation cycle. After each cycle the foil is incubated in broth for three or four days. If spores grow in the broth then clearly sterilisation was inadequate. The delay of several days before sterilisation is checked by this method is a considerable drawback to the technique.

After sterilisation, packs of instruments are kept in dust-free, dry areas. They are marked with an expiry date and used in rotation.

Ophthalmic Out-Patient Department

This is usually an area that can be readily darkened, with separate cubicles or rooms. Ideally each cubicle should have its own slit-lamp microscope, lens box, illuminated Snellen test type and set of eye drops. Multidose drop bottles of local anaesthetic, mydriatics, etc, should be changed after each clinic session. Fluorescein is provided in minims or as impregnated strips of paper (see chapter 8). A couch is required for indirect ophthalmoscopy and separate rooms should be available for testing visual fields, photography, angiography and for orthoptic examination. A treatment room is necessary for carrying out minor operations and procedures such as removing lashes (epilation), syringing the lacrimal drainage passages and subconjunctival injections. The care of patients is generally more efficient if they all have their visual acuities checked on arriving in the department. Some procedures (e.g., recording blood pressure, urinalysis, dilatation of the pupil) may usefully be performed, at a doctor's request, after he has perused the notes but before he has started examining the patient. Many patients attending eye out-patient departments are diabetic. They may require a snack if they have to wait long in the department.

Casualty

Most eye hospitals run a casualty service for those patients who simply walk into the hospital and those others referred by the General Practitioners as urgent cases. These patients may either be fitted into the work of the Out-Patient Clinic or seen separately. In those localities where such a service exists, patients with eye problems may be referred from General Accident and Emergency Departments after only a cursory examination.

The ophthalmic trained nurse working in Casualty should test the visual acuity of all patients on their arrival in the department. She should take a history and be prepared to remove both subtarsal and some corneal foreign bodies before calling the Casualty Officer. Patients with relatively minor conditions (e.g., corneal foreign bodies), should be followed up in Casualty. Patients with more serious problems should be referred to an Out-Patient Clinic or, if necessary, be admitted to hospital.

7 MICROBIOLOGY

The eye may be infected by many types of microbe (i.e., bacteria, viruses and fungi). Infections usually begin in the extraocular tissues (lids, lacrimal apparatus and conjunctiva). Once established there, they may spread to the intraocular tissues (uveal tract and retina). Intraocular infections are more difficult to treat and often cause permanent loss of sight. Thus, no eye infection should be treated lightly.

The spread of infection from extraocular to intraocular tissues is particularly likely if an operation is performed on an infected eye. Therefore, patients with lid, lacrimal sac or conjunctival infections should have their operations postponed. Some surgeons prefer cultures to be taken from the conjunctival sac pre-operatively, but a white eye rarely harbours pathogens. The routine instillation of antibiotic drops at the beginning of the operation acts as an additional safety measure.

Collection of Specimens

Conjunctival Swab

The lower fornix is swabbed with a cotton wool bud. Any infected matter that is present should be collected on to the swab.

Corneal Scrape

After the instillation of local anaesthetic drops, a speculum is inserted to hold the lids apart. The base of any corneal ulcer is gently scraped with a metal scraper.

Anterior Chamber Tap

Pus from the anterior chamber may be drawn off through a needle (paracentesis) and collected for culture (see chapter 17).

Specimens from either the conjunctiva or the cornea may be taken on the ward or in casualty or in the clinic. An anterior chamber tap is carried out in theatre. In some eye departments, doctors deal with specimens immediately by spreading them on to agar plates (for bacterial culture) or into tubes containing a tissue preparation (for virus culture). Often, however, the swabs are simply put into a transport medium and sent to the laboratory.

Specimens should be correctly taken and placed in the appropriate tubes or bottles. If necessary, a bacteriologist should be asked for advice. Specimens should be correctly labelled and accompanied by a request card on which full details are given. These should include details of any antibiotics the patient has been given. All plates and tissue cultures should be incubated immediately they have been prepared. Specimens in transport media should be sent to the laboratory immediately or, alternatively, refrigerated until the laboratory staff can deal with them.

Results of Culture

The results of cultures are usually available after twenty-four hours. Antibiotic sensitivities (i.e., which antibiotics the cultured organism is sensitive to) take forty-eight hours to be identified. The appearance of some organisms in a Gram-stained film is characteristic. Such a film can be prepared from the swab in a few minutes and may give very useful early information in an urgent case.

Cultures from the eye often grow organisms such as *Bacterium xerosis* or *Staphylococcus albus* (epidermidis). These organisms are not pathogenic to the eye and treatment with antibiotics is not required.

The bacteria most commonly cultured from infected eyes are *Staphylococcus aureus, Pneumococcus* and *Pseudomonas. Pseudomonas pyocyanea* may contaminate weak antiseptics (e.g., Cetavlon), fluorescein solutions, respirators and drains. Occasionally, several patients in a hospital develop *Pseudomonas* infections at the same time. This is a catastrophe, for *Pseudomonas* infections are difficult to treat. Patients often lose the infected eye. The antibiotics that are required are both toxic and expensive. It may be necessary to close both the operating theatre and wards until the source of infection is discovered. The bacteriologist should be asked for advice as soon as such an outbreak of infection is suspected.

8 PHARMACOLOGY

Drugs used to treat the eye may be given locally as drops (guttae), as ointment (occulentum) and as subconjunctival injections. Alternatively, they may be given systemically either by mouth or by injection. Local therapy is adequate only in the treatment of conditions of the conjunctiva, cornea and anterior uvea. Subconjunctival injections usually give a high concentration of drugs in these tissues. Systemic treatment is necessary for treating conditions of the posterior uvea, the retina and the orbit. In spite of these various approaches the penetration of some drugs within the eye is relatively poor.

Drops may be instilled into the lower fornix by asking the patient to look up and by drawing the lower lid slightly down. Alternatively, drops may be instilled by asking the patient to look down, retracting the upper lid and dropping them on to the upper sclera. This allows the drops to flow over and to diffuse through the cornea before they are washed away by the tears. Ointments are squeezed into the lower fornix. It is important not to contaminate droppers of bottles and nozzles of tubes by touching either the eye or the lids during these procedures.

Ointments prolong the contact between the drug and the tissues but patients often dislike them because they blur their vision. Ointments, therefore, are best reserved for use at bedtime.

Subconjunctival injections are given after the instillation of local anaesthetic drops and the insertion of a lid retractor. The conjunctiva of either the upper or the lower fornix is picked up with blunt forceps and the needle tip inserted through the elevated conjunctiva. The injected drug raises a bleb which usually soon disperses, although an insoluble drug like Depomedrone characteristically leaves a deposit which will be visible for several days until it is either absorbed or leaks into the conjunctival sac.

Drops should be stored in sterile glass or plastic bottles. Each ward patient should have his own set of bottles. In the clinic, drop bottles should be changed after each out-patient session. Contaminated droppers must be discarded immediately. Some drops are available in single dose, plastic minims. These avoid cross-contamination but they are expensive.

Drops are highly concentrated. One drop may contain a systemic dose of the drug. Drugs which are well absorbed (e.g., atropine) may cause systemic side effects, particularly in children and the elderly.

Many drugs have several names. One is the approved name (e.g., cyclopentolate); the others are trade names (e.g., Mydrilate). In this book approved names are used with trade names given in brackets.

Miotics (Table 8.1)

These are either cholinergic compounds or anticholinesterase inhibitors (see chapter 2). They are used to constrict the pupil, particularly in intraocular surgery and narrow-angle glaucoma and also to reverse mydriatics (chapters 16 and 17).

Common side-effects include conjunctival irritation and blurred vision due to spasm of the ciliary body.

Mydriatics (Tables 8.2 and 8.3)

These may be either cholinergic blockers or adrenergic compounds (see chapter 2). They are used to dilate the pupil prior to cataract extraction, for inspection of the fundus (fundoscopy), and to break down posterior synechiae in iritis (see chapter 15).

Many of the cholinergic blockers also cause paralysis of the ciliary body musculature (cycloplegia). This effect is an advantage for the ophthalmologist if retinoscopy is to be carried out in addition to fundoscopy. However, it is a nuisance for the patient as it causes blurring of vision due to paralysis of accommodation (chapter 2). Tropicamide and the adrenergic compounds do not cause cycloplegia.

Local side-effects include photophobia (due to dilation of the pupil) and allergic reactions of both the skin and conjunctiva. Systemic absorption may cause a fast heart beat (tachycardia).

Cycloplegics

These drugs are used to paralyse the ciliary body, to allow retinoscopy, and for the relief of pain in both keratitis and iritis (Table 8.3). They are mydriatics. Their side-effects have been discussed earlier.

Vasoconstrictors

Adrenaline is the principal vasoconstrictor used in ophthalmic surgery. It is given in the form of drops or by injection in order to reduce bleeding and to prevent dispersion of any local anaesthetic. Cocaine drops are sometimes given to potentiate the effect of adrenaline.

Table 8.1: Miotics

Approved name	Trade name	Concentration	Method of administration	Duration	Strength
acetylcholine	Miochol	1 in 5000	Anterior chamber injection	Short	Strong
pilocarpine	Isoptocarpine Sno-pilo	0.5% 1% 2% 3% 4%	Drops	Short	Strong
physostigmine	Eserine	¼%	Drops	Long	Very strong
ecothiopate iodide	Phospholine Iodide	0.03% 0.06% 0.125% 0.25%	Drops	Long	Very strong

Table 8.2: Mydriatics — Cholinergic Blockers

Approved name	Trade name	Concentration	Method of administration	Duration	Strength
atropine	— —	1% 2%	Drops Ointment	Long 10 days	Very strong
homatropine	— —	1% 2%	Drops	Long 3 days	Strong
cyclopentolate	Mydrilate	0.1% 0.5% 1%	Drops	Short 6 hours	Strong
tropicamide	Mydriacyl	0.5% 1%	Drops	Short 4 hours	Strong
hyoscine	Scopolamine	0.2%	Drops	Short	Weak
lachesine (E3)	— —	1%	Drops	Short 8 hours	Weak

Table 8.3: Mydriatics — Adrenergic Compounds

Approved name	Trade name	Concentration	Method of administration	Duration	Strength
adrenaline	Eppy	1%	Drops	12 hours	Weak
	Isoptoepinal	0.5% 1%	Drops	12 hours	Weak
	Simplene	0.5% 1%	Drops	12 hours	Weak
	Mydricaine	{ 1mg atropine 5mg cocaine 100 µg adrenaline in 0.3ml }	Sub-conjunctival	24 hours	Strong
phenylephrine		0.1% - 10%	Drops	Several hours	Weak

The absorption of adrenaline into the blood stream may cause tachycardia and cardiac arrhythmias, particularly during general anaesthesia when halothane is used. The anaesthetist's permission should always be sought before adrenaline is administered. Cocaine and adrenaline should not be given when mydriasis is undesirable (e.g., in narrow-angle glaucoma).

Drugs Lowering the Intraocular Pressure

Many different types of drugs lower the intraocular pressure and hence are useful in the treatment of glaucoma (Table 8.4). Cholinergic compounds have been used for many years although the mechanism of their action in lowering the intraocular pressure in chronic open-angle glaucoma is not well understood. The associated miosis often causes problems for the patient as it reduces the amount of light entering the eye. This may cause a reduction of vision particularly in those patients with central lens opacities.

Cholinergic drugs are also used in acute angle-closure glaucoma in the hope that by constricting the pupil the peripheral part of the iris will be pulled out of the angle.

Ecothiopate iodide is an irreversible cholinesterase inhibitor used both in treating patients with glaucoma and also in strengthening the accommodation of patients with convergent squints. It may prolong the effect of suxamethonium given during anaesthesia, thus causing prolonged apnoea. The drugs should therefore be stopped some weeks before any elective surgery. It may also cause iris cysts and cataracts.

Adrenergic compounds also cause a fall in the intraocular pressure. The associated mydriasis leads to their use being contra-indicated in narrow-angle glaucoma. (As the pupil dilates, the iris may bunch up in the angle to such an extent that the angle becomes occluded). Timolol (a β-blocker) is effective in lowering the intraocular pressure and it is well tolerated by most patients. It is very expensive. It does not affect the pupil.

Acetazolamide and dichlorphenamide reduce the production of aqueous humour by inhibiting the enzyme carbonic anhydrase (chapter 2). These drugs are used to control high intraocular pressures during the post-operative period, in the initial treatment of narrow-angle glaucoma and to supplement topical treatment in chronic open-angle glaucoma. These preparations may cause nausea, 'pins and needles' in the fingers and toes, and urinary stones. Potassium supplements are sometimes prescribed concurrently to try to lessen these complications.

Table 8.4: Drugs Lowering Intraocular Pressure

Approved name	Trade name	Types of drug	Concentration	Method of administration	Duration	Strength
pilocarpine	Isoptocarpine Sno-pilo	cholinergic compound	0.5%, 1%, 2%, 3%, 4%, 6%	Drops	Short	Strong
physostigmine	Eserine	cholinergic compound	¼-1%	Drops	Long	Very strong
ecothiopate iodide	Phospholine iodide	cholinergic compound	0.03%, 0.06%, 0.125%, 0.25%	Drops	Long	Very strong
adrenaline	Eppy Simplene Isoptoepinal	adrenergic compound	1% 0.5%, 1% 0.5%, 1%	Drops	12 hours	Weak
guanethidine	Ismelin	adrenergic compound	5%	Drops	12 hours	Weak
guanethidine + adrenaline	Ganda	adrenergic compound	3 + ½% 5 + ½% 5 + 1% 1 + 0.2%	Drops	12 hours	Weak
timolol	Timoptol	adrenergic (β) blocker	0.25%, 0.5%	Drops	12 hours	Strong
acetazolamide	Diamox	carbonic anhydrase inhibitor	250mg 500mg 500mg	Oral (Tablets) IV	6 hours	Strong
dichlorphenamide	Daranide	carbonic anhydrase inhibitor	50mg	Oral (Tablets)	6 hours	Strong
glycerol		osmotic diuretics	Dose IG/kg body weight	Oral (Liquid)	Short	Strong
mannitol		osmotic diuretics	20% solution	IV	Short	Strong

Local Anaesthetics (Table 8.5)

Anaesthetic drops may be used to numb the conjunctiva and cornea for minor procedures such as applanation tonometry, removal of superficial foreign bodies, corneal scraping, iodisation and removal of corneal sutures. Several drops are often necessary. The lid margins are also slightly numbed, which is useful when epilation and lacrimal probing are to be carried out. Local anaesthetic drops are used in conjunction with both infiltration of the skin and nerve blocks when more major procedures are planned. The eye remains anaesthetised for some time after the instillation of the drops. Ideally, therefore, the eye should be padded to protect it from trauma, such as might be sustained were a foreign body to lodge on the cornea.

Clearly, carrying out procedures under local anaesthesia on both eyes simultaneously raises the question as to whether both eyes should be padded. This completely incapacitates the patient. Thus, when both eyes require such treatment, it may be judged necessary to carry out treatment first on one eye and then on the other.

Local anaesthetics may damage the corneal epithelium and hence delay healing of a corneal abrasion. They should not, therefore, be used routinely to prevent pain from an abrasion, although their use to secure a good view of the eye may be invaluable.

Almost any ophthalmic operation may be performed under local anaesthesia. Usually a facial nerve block is given in order to paralyse the muscles with which the patient closes the eye. The injection site overlies the neck of the mandible. The surgeon locates this by asking the patient to open and close his mouth while he himself feels in front of the patient's ear.

A retrobulbar injection is given in order to block the ciliary ganglion and thus complete the anaesthesia of the globe. The injection site is at the lower outer corner of the orbit. The patient is asked to look slightly upwards and inwards whilst the injection is given. This helps the surgeon to place the tip of the needle in the correct position. The needle should be inserted initially straight backwards and then towards the apex of the orbit to a depth of about 3 cm. The lids and superior rectus insertion may be infiltrated prior to the insertion of traction sutures. No more than twenty millilitres of 1 per cent lignocaine should be injected. A greater dose may lead to the patient developing convulsions.

Table 8.5: Local Anaesthetics

Approved name	Trade name	Concentration	Method of administration	Strength
oxybuprocaine	Benoxinate	0.4%	Drops	Weak
amethocaine	Pantocaine	0.5% 1%	Drops	Strong
proxymetacaine	Ophthaine	0.5%	Drops	Weak
cocaine		2% 4%	Drops	Strong
lignocaine	Xylocaine	0.5% 1% 1.5% 2%	Infiltration	Strong
procaine		2%	Infiltration	Strong

Table 8.6: Antibiotics

Approved name	Trade name	Concentration	Method of administration
chloramphenicol	Chloromycetin	0.5% 1%	Drops Ointment
penicillin G		2500 units/ml Dose 1,000,000 units Daily	Drops IV or IM
neomycin		0.5%	Drops
gentamycin	Genticin	0.3% (15% concentrated) 20mg in 0.5 ml 80mg t.i.d.	Drops Subconjunctival IV
sulphacetamide	Albucid	10%, 20%, 30% 2.5%	Drops Ointment
framycetin	Soframycin	0.5% 0.5%	Drops Ointment
polymixin bacitracin	Polyfax	10,000 units per g 500 units per g	Ointment
ampicillin	Penbritin	Dose 250-500 mg q.i.d.	Oral or IV
sodium fusidate	Fucidin	Dose 500 mg t.i.d.	Oral
methicillin	Celbenin	500 mg in 0.5ml Dose IG q.i.d.	Subconjunctival IV
tetracycline	Achromycin	250 mg	Tablets
chlortetracycline cephaloridine	Aureomycin Ceporin	1% 50 mg in 0.5ml Dose 1-2G daily	Ointment Subconjunctival IV

Antibiotics (Table 8.6)

For local treatment, broad spectrum antibiotics are chosen. They quite often induce allergic skin reactions. Chloramphenicol is frequently prescribed because it is effective, cheap and well tolerated. Penicillin drops should be prepared just prior to their use. Penicillin is usually reserved for treating patients with gonococcal ophthalmia (chapter 12). Antibiotic drops need to be given frequently; hourly in severe infections, four times daily in mild ones.

Gentamycin is very useful as a subconjunctival injection, for a large amount of the drug can be dissolved in a small volume of solvent. When systemic antibiotics are required they are chosen according to the sensitivity of the infecting organism. When this is not known a broad spectrum antibiotic or a mixture of drugs is given.

Antiviral Agents (Table 8.7)

These are used mainly in the treatment of Herpes simplex keratitis. They are given at least five times daily for ten days. They may cause corneal erosions or occlusion of the lacrimal puncta. They should not be given to pregnant women.

Antifungal Agents (Table 8.8)

These are all irritants to the eye and they may cause toxic effects. Usually a combination of drugs is most effective in treating fungal infections, but even so treatment may be unsuccessful.

Table 8.7: Antiviral Agents

Approved name	Trade name	Concentration	Method of administration
idoxuridine	Dendrid	0.1%	Drops
	Kerecid	0.1% 0.5%	Drops Ointment
vidarabine	Vira-A	3%	Ointment
trifluorothymidine (F_3T)		1%	Drops
acycloguanosine		3%	Ointment
acyclovir	Zovirax	3% 200 mg	Ointment Tablets

Table 8.8: Antifungal Agents

Approved name	Trade name	Concentration	Method of administration
nystatin		1%	Drops
amphotericin	Fungizone	5% Dose up to 1.5 mg daily	Ointment IV or subconjunctival
pimaricin	Natamycin	5% 1%	Drops Ointment
tobramycin	Tobralex	0.3%	Drops

Anti-inflammatory Agents (Table 8.9)

These drugs are used in allergic conjunctivitis, uveitis and in severe infections — in conjunction with antibiotics (see chapter 17). Combined preparations of a steroid and an antibiotic (e.g., Betnesol N) are useful in post-operative uveitis and blepharitis.

Local steroids may aggravate *Herpes simplex* keratitis and, in addition, cause cataracts and glaucoma. Oral steroids may aggravate pulmonary tuberculosis, peptic ulceration and diabetes. Patients on oral steroids should carry blue warning cards.

Table 8.9: Anti-inflammatory Agents

Approved name	Trade name	Concentration	Method of administration	Strength
prednisolone	Predsol	0.5% (0.3%, 0.1%, 0.05%, 0.03%, 0.001%, 0.003%). Dose up to 100mg daily	Drops Tabs	Weak
betamethasone	Betnesol	0.1% 0.1% 4mg in 1ml	Drops Ointment Subconjunctival	Strong
dexamethasone	Maxidex	0.1%	Drops	Very Strong
methyl- prednisolone	Depomedrone	40mg in 1ml	Drops	Very Strong

Staining Agents

Fluorescein is an orange dye. When diluted it becomes green and shows up well in blue light. In the conjunctival sac it stains ulcers, corneal abrasions and the tear film. It is used in applanation tonometry and in carrying out Seidel's test (see chapter 17). It is injected intravenously as a 20 per cent solution during angiography (see chapter 19).

Fluorescein solution favours the growth of *Pseudomonas aeruginosa*. For this reason the dye should be supplied only in minims (as 2 per cent solution) or as impregnated strips of paper, and never in standard drop bottles. Outbreaks of *Pseudomonas* infection have been due to the use of contaminated fluorescein solutions.

Fluorescein damages soft contact lenses. Such lenses should not be re-inserted for several hours after the dye's instillation.

Rose bengal (1 per cent drops) is a red dye which shows up best in green light. It stains dying cells and mucus and it is useful in the diagnosis of dry eyes (chapter 11). Its use in examining patients with dry eyes may cause severe pain and such examinations should be kept to the absolute minimum.

Miscellaneous Drugs

Artificial tears such as Hypromellose, BJ6 and Tears Naturale are used in kerato-conjunctivitis sicca (chapter 11).

Xylometazoline/antazoline (Otrivine-Antistine) drops are useful in mild allergic conjunctivitis.

Zinc sulphate and adrenaline drops are used for treating watering eyes when surgery is inadvisable.

Carbolic acid/iodine solution is used for treating dendritic ulcers (chapter 13).

70 per cent Alcohol may be used as a retrobulbar injection to relieve pain in a sightless eye (chapter 16).

Alpha chymotrypsin (Zonulysin) 0.5 ml of 1 in 5000 solution is injected into the posterior chamber prior to intracapsular cataract extraction (chapter 17).

Normal saline may be used to irrigate either the conjunctival sac or the anterior chamber (chapter 23 and 17).

Glycerine drops are used prior to gonioscopy if the patient has corneal oedema.

Methylcellulose (Methocel) is a viscous solution used when either a gonioscope or a fundus contact lens is applied to the eye.

PART TWO

DISEASES AND THEIR TREATMENT

9 ORBIT

Introduction

The orbits lie either side of the nasal cavity and contain the eyes and their associated structures. The orbital margins in front are strong and serve to protect the eyes from injury. The walls of the orbit are thin and are readily fractured.

Any increase in the volume of the orbital contents leads to forward displacement of the eye which is often accompanied by protrusion of the lids. This displacement may be directly forward (axial) or eccentric. Such eccentric displacement of the globe indicates the site of the lesion (Figure 9.1) and the rate of displacement gives a clue to the lesion's pathology.

Proptosis is assessed by comparing the position of one eye with that of the other and also by assessing its relationship to that of the orbital margins. More precise measurements may be made with an exophthalmometer.

The growth of the orbit is proportional to the growth of the eye. Whereas the orbit of a child with a distended eye (e.g., buphthalmos) will be large, that containing a little (e.g., microphthalmic) eye will be small. The orbits may be underdeveloped in various congenital anomalies of the skull, so that the eyes appear prominent.

Figure 9.1: Eccentric Displacement Due to Lacrimal Gland Tumour

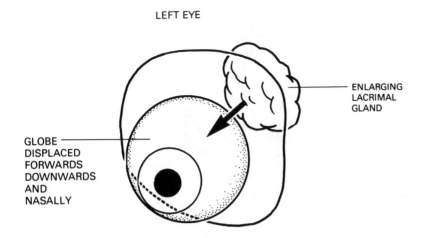

LEFT EYE

ENLARGING
LACRIMAL
GLAND

GLOBE
DISPLACED
FORWARDS
DOWNWARDS
AND
NASALLY

Acute Infection or Orbital Cellulitis

Infection commonly spreads from the adjacent paranasal air sinuses (Figure 9.2) or more rarely, by septic emboli from a distant site. In early childhood the medial wall of the orbit is membranous and organisms can easily spread from infected ethmoidal air cells.

Signs and Symptoms

The patient feels ill and there may be severe pain around the eye. Double vision (due to displacement of the eye) may be noted if the swollen upper lid is lifted.

The conjunctiva is oedematous and the blood vessels engorged. The proptosed eye may be immobile (ophthalmoplegia) and examination of the fundus may show the retinal veins to be distended. A fluctuant abscess may develop which presents most commonly at the upper and inner aspect of the orbit.

Figure 9.2: Orbital Cellulitis — Spread of Infection from Nasal Sinuses

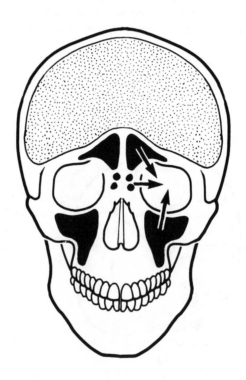

Complications

Serious complications may arise which threaten the patient's life as well as his sight. They include, exposure keratitis, visual loss due to optic nerve damage, meningitis and cavernous sinus thrombosis.

Treatment

Initially, full doses of appropriate antibiotics should be given systemically. The opinion of an ear, nose and throat surgeon should be sought urgently. Local heat will help to alleviate pain and treatment should be given for any underlying condition (e.g., sinusitis). Any abscess should be drained.

Chronic Infection and Pseudotumour

The time-honoured causes of chronic infection, leading to granuloma formation, namely syphilis and tuberculosis, are now rare. However, a similar clinical picture of painful proptosis associated with diplopia is not uncommon. The cause of such an orbital pseudotumour is often not discovered. The blood supply to the optic nerve is always at risk and sudden blindness may ensue. High doses of systemic steroids may alleviate the condition.

Carotico-cavernous Fistula

Such a fistula may result either from an injury or from spontaneous rupture of a carotid aneurysm into the cavernous sinus. Arterial blood under high pressure enters the venous sinus and passes into the veins of the orbit. The raised pressure in the veins results in oedema of the lids and of the conjunctiva (chemosis) and the eye is pushed forwards. The arterial pulsation is transmitted to the eye causing pulsating exophthalmos. A pulsatile noise, a bruit, may be heard when a stethoscope is placed over the orbit. Both eyes may be involved because of the venous communications between the cavernous sinuses. This is sometimes a painful condition, with loss of vision due to embarrassment of the blood supply to the optic nerve or to corneal exposure or secondary glaucoma. Treatment by ligating the internal carotid artery may be considered but the risk of precipitating a hemiplegia due to cerebral ischaemia needs to be carefully assessed.

Retrobulbar Haemorrhage

Bleeding within the orbit may result from trauma or follow a retrobulbar injection being given. The proptosis subsides spontaneously but the raised pressure within the orbit may damage the optic nerve. Any planned intraocular operation should be postponed until the haemorrhage has been absorbed.

Tumours and Non-tumour Masses

Displacement of the eye may indicate the presence of an orbital tumour but inflammatory conditions or a disordered thyroid (chapter 22) are more likely causes. Tumours may involve the orbit in the following ways:

1. A primary tumour, either benign or malignant, may arise from any of the tissues normally found within the orbit.
2. A secondary deposit (metastasis) may arise from a remote primary lesion.
3. Invasion by a malignant tumour arising from a nearby structure.

Primary Tumours

These include tumours of the lacrimal gland, haemangioma, optic nerve glioma, meningioma and rhabdomyosarcoma.

Signs and Symptoms

These vary with the type of tumour. They may include proptosis, pain, visual loss due to optic nerve compression, squint and diplopia.

Special Investigations

These include X-rays of the orbit and optic foramen, biopsy, orbital venography and carotid angiography. Ultrasound examination and computerised axial tomography (CT scan) may provide very helpful information.

Metastatic Orbital Tumours

Such tumours most commonly arise from primary bronchial carcinoma in men, breast carcinoma in women and nephroblastoma in children, or from lymphoreticular tumours.

Secondary Orbital Tumours

There may be invasive spread from tumours of the eyelids, conjunctiva, globe, paranasal air sinuses or cranial cavity. The signs and symptoms that arise are those of the underlying condition in addition to the proptosis.

Treatment of Orbital Tumours

Treatment varies depending upon the size of the lesion, its likely pathology and whether there is involvement of other structures. Possibilities include orbitotomy and local excision, irradiation and removal of the entire orbital contents (exenteration).

Non-Tumour Masses

These may mimic orbital tumours by causing proptosis, but they are not true neoplasms.

Dermoid Cysts

These are congenital in origin but they may present in adult life. They most commonly arise at the upper outer angle of the orbit. Their cheesy contents consist of epithelial cells, fat and sometimes hairs. Treatment by excision may be difficult because of either extension of the cyst into the depths of the orbit or communication through a bony defect with the cranial cavity.

Orbital Varix

This is a congenital venous malformation. Proptosis may be intermittent, appearing only when there is venous back pressure in the orbit, which becomes apparent when the patient either lowers his head or blows his nose. Orbital venography is diagnostic. Excision of a varix is rarely indicated.

10 LIDS

For details of the relevant anatomy and physiology, see chapter 2.

Inflammation

Squamous Blepharitis

Inflammation of the lid margins is a common, chronic condition. The patient complains of sore eyes and the lid margins are red, thickened and scaly. Such patients often have dandruff. Treatment consists of regular cleaning of the lash roots with removal of any crusts and grease and the application of an antibiotic ointment. Steroid-antibiotic ointments are helpful but should be given only under ophthalmic supervision for their prolonged use may cause unsightly atrophy of the skin of the lids.

Ulcerative Blepharitis

In severe blepharitis there may be ulceration of the lid margins due to infection with bacteria such as *Staphylococcus aureus.* The lids are red, painful and ulcerated and discharge pus. Conjunctivitis is a usual accompaniment. Intensive antibiotic treatment with drops and ointment is required.

Herpes Simplex

Infection with this virus may cause painful sores on the eyelids. Sometimes both lid and corneal lesions appear together so that the eye itself should be closely examined. Lid lesions heal spontaneously in about ten days but treatment with an antiviral ointment is advisable to prevent spread of the virus to the eye.

Herpes Zoster

See chapter 13.

Stye

This is an infection of an eyelash follicle (Figure 10.1). There is initially a small patch of inflammation which resolves when a bead of pus discharges on the lid margin. An antibiotic ointment may be applied to prevent any spread of infection. Recurrent styes may be due to chronic blepharitis or associated with diabetes.

Chalazion (Meibomian Cyst)

This is an infection of a Meibomian gland (Figure 10.2). The patient complains of a red, tender swelling in the lid. With hot bathing and treatment with an

Figure 10.1: Stye

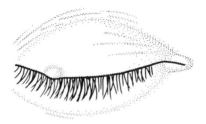

antibiotic ointment this may completely resolve. Occasionally the gland discharges pus through the surface of the skin. Often, however, a small swelling persists. The cyst may be uncomfortable, unsightly or distort vision due to pressure on the globe. Such impaired vision is especially likely if the chalazion is in the centre of the upper lid.

Figure 10.2: Meibomian Cyst

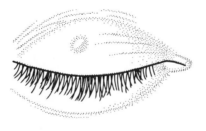

Persistent chalazia are treated with incision and curettage (I & C). Anaesthetic drops are instilled and a local anaesthetic injected around the chalazion. The needle should pass deep to the orbicularis muscle to lie between the muscle and the tarsal plate. It is in this plane that the nerves and vessels lie. A chalazion clamp is applied and the lid is everted. A vertical incision is made through the tarsal plate and the contents of the chalazion are scraped out with a curette (Figure 10.3). Care should be taken not to damage the lid margin or the lacrimal punctum. If pus is released curettage is not necessary. An antibiotic ointment is applied and the clamp is removed. The eye is held closed with a pad and bandage. The patient may return home soon afterwards, removing the dressing next day and applying ointment three times a day for a week.

Figure 10.3: Incision and Curettage

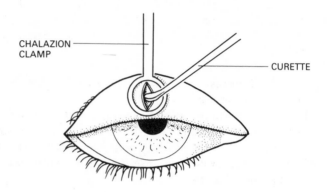

CHALAZION
CLAMP

CURETTE

Lid Cysts

Cysts of Moll and Zeiss are small retention cysts that commonly occur at the lid margin. The former are transluscent and are filled with watery fluid. The latter are yellowish and contain sebaceous material. If unsightly, they may be deroofed and their contents evacuated under local anaesthesia.

Lid Malposition

Ptosis

This is a drooping of the upper lid. Causes include:

1. Congenital. Underdevelopment of the levator palpebrae superioris muscle.
2. Mechanical. The lid is too heavy because of either inflammation or thickening.
3. Muscle diseases, e.g., myasthenia gravis, dystrophia myotonica or senility.
4. Oculomotor (third cranial nerve) palsy.
5. Lesion of the sympathetic pathways (Horner's syndrome).
6. Injury to the levator muscle (chapter 23).

Signs and Symptoms. The eye is either partially or totally closed. In a child, amblyopia may develop if the lid covers the pupillary area virtually all the time. Amblyopia may not develop in some children whose pupil is occluded when they look straight ahead, if the pupil is uncovered when they look down. The patient may wrinkle up his forehead and tilt his head back in an attempt to improve his vision.

Treatment. Some cases improve spontaneously (e.g., third nerve palsy). Patients with myasthenia may improve with the use of anticholinesterase drugs. Patients with muscle disorders are best treated with lid props placed on either spectacles or contact lenses. Mild cases of senile and congenital origin are best left alone.

Severe congenital cases may be treated by resection of the levator muscle through the skin (Everbush's operation) or through the conjunctiva (Blaskovic's operation), or, alternatively, by a fascia lata sling connecting the lid to the muscles of the forehead. Severe senile ptosis may be treated by resection of a small length of the levator muscle together with a strip of the adjacent tarsal plate (Fascanella's operation). Surgical overcorrection of ptosis may be followed by exposure of the cornea which in turn may cause impairment of vision.

Ectropion

This means that the lid margin turns outwards. It usually affects the lower lid. It may be due to senile laxity of the orbicularis muscle or to skin scarring following burns (cicatricial ectropion). Tears pool behind the everted lid and then spill out so that the patient's chief complaint is of epiphora. The inevitable constant wiping of the eye may worsen the condition unless the patient can be taught to wipe the eye upwards and inwards.

Senile cases may be treated with excision of wedges of the skin and tarsal plate (wedge resection, Kuhnt Zymanowski's operation) (Figure 10.4). In very mild cases application of a cautery just behind the punctum, which causes conjunctival scarring, may suffice to draw the lid back against the eye (Figure 10.5).

Entropion

In this common condition, the lid margin turns inwards. Senile entropion is due to laxity of the tissues of the lower lid, so allowing part of the orbicularis muscle to ride up over the lid margin and turn the lashes inwards (Figure 10.6). Cicatricial entropion is due to conjunctival scarring as a result of burns or trachoma (chapter 12). Entropion may affect either the upper or lower lid. The inturned lashes abrade both the conjunctiva and cornea causing redness, discharge and the sensation of a foreign body being in the eye. Secondary infection and corneal scarring, with loss of vision, may result. Prompt treatment is necessary. As a temporary measure an antibiotic ointment should be applied and a strip of adhesive tape placed on the lid and on the adjacent cheek so that the lashes are held away from the eye. Later an operation should be performed.

Figure 10.4: Kuhnt Zymanowski's Operation

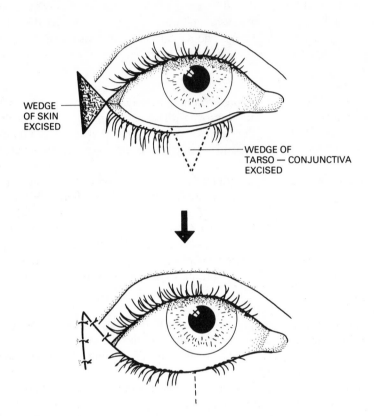

WEDGE
OF SKIN
EXCISED

WEDGE OF
TARSO — CONJUNCTIVA
EXCISED

Figure 10.5: Retropunctal Cautery

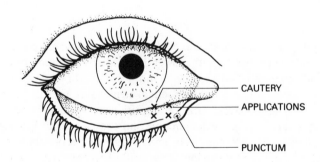

CAUTERY

APPLICATIONS

PUNCTUM

Figure 10.6: Senile Entropion

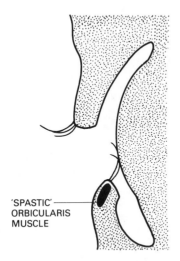

'SPASTIC'
ORBICULARIS
MUSCLE

Operations for senile entropion include:

a) Skin and muscle operation (Figure 10.7). A strip of orbicularis muscle and the overlying skin is excised.
b) Wheeler's operation (Figure 10.8). A strip of orbicularis muscle is isolated and part of it is excised. The ends are joined and sutured to the tarsal plate. This prevents the muscle riding up over the lid margin and consequently everting it.
c) Weis's operation (Figure 10.9). A full thickness incision is made through the lower lid. Sutures are inserted as shown and tightened until the lid margin is slightly everted.

Cicatricial entropion may be corrected by Kettersey's operation (Figure 10.10).

Trichiasis

This term is used when the lashes are inturned whilst the lid margin remains in a normal position. It may be congenital in origin or follow trauma, burns or trachoma. It causes the same problems as entropion. Plucking out the lashes (epilation) brings temporary relief, but treatment entails destruction of the eyelash follicles by either electrolysis or cryotherapy. Alternatively, an operation to evert the lid margin may be preferable.

Figure 10.7: Skin and Muscle Operation

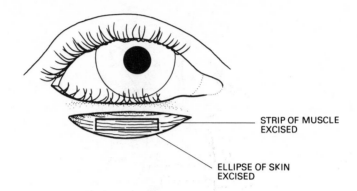

STRIP OF MUSCLE
EXCISED

ELLIPSE OF SKIN
EXCISED

Figure 10.8: Wheeler's Operation

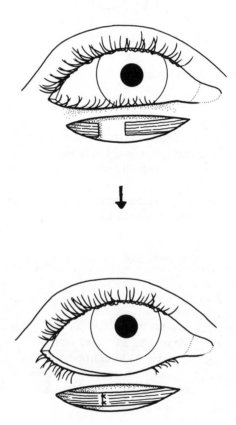

Figure 10.9: Weis's Operation

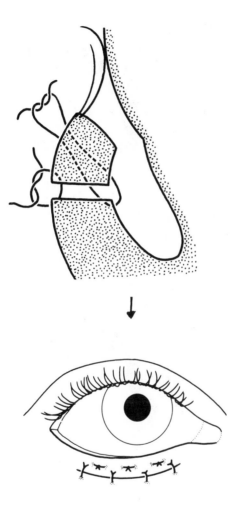

Electrolysis. This is best performed under the microscope. Anaesthetic drops are instilled and a local anaesthetic is injected into the lid margin around the offending lashes. For safety a haptic contact lens may be used to protect the eye. The anode plate electrode is strapped to the arm after the application of an electrode jelly. The cathode needle electrode is inserted deeply into the lash follicle and the current turned on until the surrounding lid turns white and the lash can be readily removed. Electrolysis is useful only in mild cases of trichiasis. It is easy to miss small lashes which may be a potent source of discomfort.

Figure 10.10: Kettersey's Operation

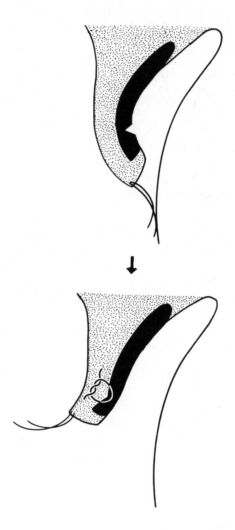

Benign Lid Tumours

Xanthelasmata

These are flat yellowish deposits within the skin. They may be due to hypercholesterolaemia which should be treated with diet or drugs. Unsightly lesions may be excised.

Neurofibromata

These vary in size from small skin lesions to huge disfiguring masses in the lids. The patient usually has other signs of neurofibromatosis (Von Recklinghausen's disease) including café-au-lait spots and skin tumours elsewhere.

Sturge-Weber Syndrome

The purple lesions of a port wine stain on the eyelids are obvious and unsightly. Advice about make-up or laser treatment may be appropriate. Vascular malformations may also occur in the angle of the anterior chamber causing glaucoma. Similar lesions may occur on the brain and may be associated with fits.

Malignant Tumours

Basal Cell Carcinoma (Rodent Ulcer)

This is a relatively common tumour of the eyelids of elderly white-skinned people who have been exposed to much sunlight. A typical rodent ulcer has a raised pearly edge, surrounding a central ulcer which may bleed. Untreated, it extends into the surrounding skin and deeper tissues and may eventually become a hideous fungating mass destroying much of the face. It never spreads to distant organs. The diagnosis should be confirmed by biopsy. Wide excision of the neoplasm with a plastic repair of the eyelids is often required. Radiotherapy is an alternative form of treatment but scarring of the skin and the conjunctiva may result and the lacrimal canaliculi may be occluded. The eye itself should be shielded with a lead contact lens for blinding complications can arise from the eye being inadvertently exposed to radiation.

Squamous Cell Carcinoma

This is a much rarer tumour. It may metastasise. Biopsy, followed by wide excision, with or without radiotherapy, is the treatment of choice.

LACRIMAL APPARATUS

The production and drainage of tears are delicately balanced in order to provide a tear film of an ideal thickness and consistency. A deficiency of tears may threaten the patient's eyesight. An excess of tears may obscure his vision or predispose to conjunctival infection. The skin of the lids and cheek may become wet and excoriated. An over-secretion of tears, due to reflex irritation of the trigeminal nerve (e.g., by a foreign body) or emotional causes is called lacrimation. The term epiphora is used when the eye waters because of poor drainage of tears due to ectropion of the lower lid or obstruction of the drainage channels.

Lacrimal Gland

Acute Dacryoadenitis

An acute infection of the lacrimal gland may develop secondary to conjunctivitis or be due to systemic diseases such as mumps or gonorrhoea. An inflamed, tender swelling develops in the upper and outer part of the orbit and upper lid causing the lid margin to assume an S-shaped curve. The patient, often a child, is unwell and febrile. Treatment is with systemic antibiotics.

Chronic Dacryoadenitis

Chronic infection of the gland may be due to tuberculosis, syphilis or sarcoidosis; often the cause is unknown. It may be accompanied by enlargement of the salivary glands in which case the term 'Mikulicz syndrome' is sometimes used. The involved glands are enlarged, firm and lobulated but they are not tender. Treatment is that of the cause.

Dry Eyes (Kerato-conjunctivitis Sicca — KCS)

An under-secretion of tears may be due to lacrimal gland disease (e.g., sarcoidosis), drugs (e.g., atropine, practolol) or conjunctival scarring — which blocks the lacrimal ductules. Patients with systemic disorders such as rheumatoid arthritis or systemic lupus erythematosis commonly suffer from dryness of the eyes; if they also have dry mouths and are arthritic they are said to have Sjögren's syndrome.

Signs and Symptoms. The eyes are dry, irritable and uncomfortable; patients often complain of a burning sensation. The eyes appear inflamed and slit-lamp microscopy shows an inadequate tear film; after Rose Bengal drops have been instilled, punctate staining of the conjunctiva and cornea may be revealed. An excess of stringy mucus may be seen in the fornices or adhering to the cornea (filamentary keratitis). When filaments are dislodged the corneal epithelium is breached, so causing painful abrasions.

Schirmer's Test. The tear secretion may be measured by placing special strips of filter paper in the lower fornices for five minutes (Figure 11.1 and Figure 11.2). The length of paper moistened with tears during this time gives an indication of the tear secretion. Normally, the strips are moistened for at least 15mm of their length. If less than 5mm are wet, then the patient definitely has dry eyes. This test should be performed before any local anaesthetic drops are instilled (e.g., for tonometry) as their presence invalidates the test. The strips should not touch the cornea as this causes reflex lacrimation. The patient may have his eyes either open or closed during the test.

Figure 11.1: Schirmer Test Strip

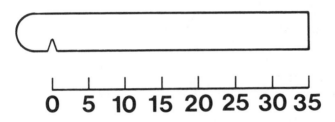

0 5 10 15 20 25 30 35

MEASURE FROM INDENTATION

Complications. Any deficiency of tears predisposes to conjunctivitis and corneal ulceration. A corneal ulcer may lead to scarring or even to perforation of the eye and hence to panophthalmitis. These complications will clearly have disastrous effects upon the patient's vision.

Management. The care of the patient with dry eyes includes thorough investigation to try to discover an underlying systemic cause. Drugs such as Practolol should be discontinued. The patient should be asked to instil artificial tears frequently (chapter 8) and perhaps use mucolytics (e.g., acetylcysteine drops) to dissolve stringy mucus. All four puncta may be sealed with the cautery so eliminating the drainage of tears and allowing their conservation. This procedure is indicated if the patient experiences relief of symptoms after a trial of occlusion of the puncta with gelatin plugs. Antibiotic drops should be prescribed in severe cases to lessen the risk of infection.

Figure 11.2: Schirmer's Test

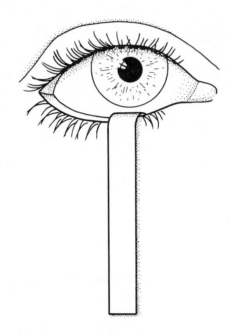

Lacrimal Gland Tumours

These may be benign (pleomorphic adenoma) or malignant (adenoid cystic carcinoma, adenocarcinoma or lymphoid tumour). A hard swelling develops. The eye is pushed downward, nasally and forwards and the patient may complain of diplopia.

Malignant tumours spread locally, through bone into the cranial cavity. The prognosis is poor. Treatment is by excision of the entire gland. Preliminary biopsy predisposes to spread of tumour cells and is thus best avoided. If local spread has occurred exenteration may be required. Radiotherapy is reserved for tumours which are too far advanced to be cured by surgery.

Lacrimal Puncta

Congenital anomalies, such as re-duplication of the puncta and canaliculi, rarely cause symptoms. Closure of the lower punctum, with resulting epiphora, may complicate herpetic eye infections or its treatment with idoxuridine. A cure may be effected by a 'one-snip' operation, in which the punctum is first dilated and then the vertical part of the lower canaliculus is incised with scissors (Figure 11.3). Eversion (ectropion) of the lower punctum causes epiphora. Treatment of the ectropion by retro-punctal cautery or wedge excision of part of the lid should relieve this.

Figure 11.3: One-snip Operation

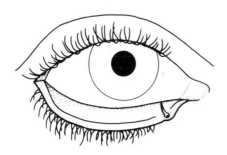

Lacrimal Canaliculi

Infection by '*Streptothrix*' (*Actinomyces*) results in chronic epiphora and a cheesy yellow discharge. It may prove necessary to slit open the infected canaliculus in order to scrape out the fungal mass.

Irradiation may cause permanent fibrosis and narrowing of the canaliculi. The stenosis may be treated by direct excision of the obstruction and anastomosis of the canaliculi with the lacrimal sac. Alternatively, intubation of the canaliculi with silicone tubes may be carried out and the tubes left in place for some months. Finally, a glass tube, designed by Lester Jones, may be inserted from the medial part of the conjunctival sac directly into the lacrimal sac thus by-passing the canaliculi. Each of these methods should be combined with a dacryocystorhinostomy. The first method is technically difficult; the second uncertain of success and the third unpopular with patients as the glass tube often irritates the eye or becomes blocked or even falls out.

Lacrimal Sac

Infection of the lacrimal sac usually occurs as a result of obstruction of the naso-lacrimal duct. The characteristically chronic infection leads to the patient having a persistently watering and discharging eye.

Acute Infection (Dacryocystitis)

This very painful condition develops over a few hours and leads to the patient feeling very unwell. There is a painful red swelling at the medial canthus usually associated with epiphora. Initially, local and systemic antibiotics are given. Incision of the pus-filled sac, or its spontaneous perforation, may bring about a more rapid resolution of the infection. However, such release of pus may lead to a lacrimal fistula developing. After an acute attack, recurrent infections are usual and the sac wall often becomes shrunken and fibrosed. Sometimes the sac remains distended, and fills with mucus, causing a mucocele. The mucus can be expressed through the puncta by pressure on the swelling. In either case a dacryocystorhinostomy (DCR) is advisable (see p.97). If the patient is unfit for a DCR, then simple excision of the sac (dacryocystectomy) may well rid the patient of the chronic discharge. Such persistent infection is always liable to cause corneal ulceration. Tear secretion in the very elderly is usually reduced and may be insufficient for epiphora to be a problem even when the nasolacrimal duct is blocked.

Nasolacrimal Duct

Congenital Obstruction

This is common in the newborn because the lower end of the duct often fails to canalise. This leads to watering of the eye and stickiness due to infection. The stickiness may be apparent at birth although often it only becomes manifest some time later. Watering of the eye is usually delayed until the baby is some weeks old because early in life few tears are produced. Occasionally, acute dacryocystitis supervenes. Frequently the duct canalises spontaneously and the condition resolves. The initial treatment is to keep the eye clean and to instil antibiotic drops regularly. The child's mother should be instructed to press gently over the lacrimal sac several times a day for although this will lead to most of the mucus regurgitating through the lower punctum, some may be forced downwards through the obstruction in the duct.

If the eye is still watering excessively at one year of age, probing under general anaesthesia is advisable. This may be done as a day case. Either the upper or lower punctum is dilated and a fine probe (00) passed first vertically and then horizontally along the canaliculus. The probe is then turned vertically downwards to pass down through the nasolacrimal duct until the bony floor of the nose is encountered. This manoeuvre disrupts the membranous obstruction present at the lower end of the duct. The duct is then syringed with air (saline might enter the child's trachea and cause respiratory problems). If, despite this operation, epiphora persists, then a second probing may be performed. If this, in turn, fails, a dacryocystorhinostomy may be necessary but this should be postponed until the child is of school age.

Acquired Obstruction

This is a common condition in the middle-aged and elderly. The patient complains of watering of the eye which may be so severe that it interferes with reading and causes changes of the skin around the eye. Acute or chronic infection may supervene.

The diagnosis may be confirmed by gently syringing the duct. Local anaesthetic drops are instilled. The lower punctum is dilated with a Nettleship's punctum dilator. Saline is injected into the lower canaliculus by using a syringe and lacrimal cannula. If the duct is blocked, saline regurgitates through both upper and lower canaliculi and the patient does not feel or taste the salt solution in his nasopharynx.

Dacryocystography (DCG). This radiological examination of the lacrimal passages is performed by syringing them with a radio opaque solution. It is helpful in establishing the site of obstruction in atypical cases.

Management. In adults probing is inappropriate and syringing is of limited value. Those patients who are elderly or unfit, for whom surgery is contra-indicated, can usually be kept comfortable by the use of astringent drops (zinc sulphate and adrenaline) together with antibiotic drops if there are signs of infection. The usual decline of lacrimal secretion with increasing age leads to patients' symptoms tending to lessen with the passage of time.

Permanent relief of symptoms is provided by a successful dacryocystorhinostomy (DCR). This operation is usually performed under general anaesthesia. The lacrimal sac is surrounded by a venous plexus and bleeding can be a problem. Bleeding is lessened by tilting the patient so that his head is uppermost. A hypotensive anaesthetic contributes to haemostasis. After protecting the cornea with a shell and packing the nose with adrenaline-soaked gauze, an incision is made close to the medial canthus and the lacrimal sac is exposed. The bony wall of the lacrimal fossa is removed with bone nibblers and the sac anastomosed to the adjacent nasal mucosa (Figure 11.4). The obstructed nasolacrimal duct is thus by-passed and tears drain unhindered into the nose. Sometimes silicone tubes are inserted to keep the canaliculi and anastomosis open whilst healing occurs. Post-operatively, local antibiotics are instilled in the eye and the patient kept in hospital for a few days. Skin stitches are removed after five days and the silicone tubes withdrawn several months later (Figure 11.5).

Figure 11.4: Dacryocystorhinostomy (DCR)

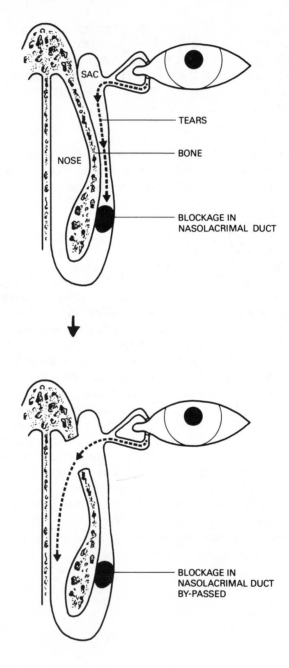

Figure 11.5: Removal of Silicone Tubes after DCR

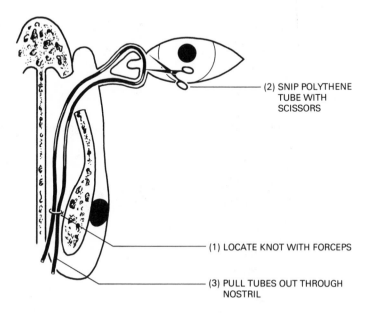

(2) SNIP POLYTHENE TUBE WITH SCISSORS

(1) LOCATE KNOT WITH FORCEPS

(3) PULL TUBES OUT THROUGH NOSTRIL

12 CONJUNCTIVA

For details of relevant anatomy and physiology, see chapter 2.

Inflammation (Conjunctivitis)

This may be acute or chronic and be due to infections, allergies or unknown causes.

Bacterial Conjunctivitis

This is commonly caused by *Staphylococcus aureus*. Other causative organisms include *Streptococci*, *Pneumococci*, *Gonococci* and *Haemophilus*.

Symptoms and Signs. Usually both eyes are affected. They feel sore and gritty and discharge purulent secretions. This tends to glue the eyelashes together overnight so that the patient has difficulty in opening his eyes in the morning. There may be slight photophobia and transient blurring of vision, especially if collections of discharge cover the cornea. The conjunctiva is red and thickened and discharge may be seen on the lashes and at the inner and outer canthi.

Complications. Corneal ulcers may develop, particularly if there is trauma to the cornea during an episode of conjunctivitis.

Treatment. Antibiotic drops are given hourly in severe cases and four times daily in milder ones. Antibiotic ointment, applied at night, lessens the stickiness in the morning. A seven-day course of treatment is usually sufficient to effect a cure. Bacterial cultures are necessary only in problem cases (chapter 7), as most patients respond to treatment with a broad spectrum antibiotic, e.g., chloramphenicol. Conjunctivitis is infectious and patients should be warned to keep their face-cloths and towels separate from those of the rest of the family and to wash their hands after touching their lids.

Ophthalmia Neonatorum

This is conjunctivitis occurring in a baby within three weeks of birth. It is a notifiable disease. The infant becomes infected by organisms in the mother's vaginal secretions. Infection may be caused by the gonococcus or chlamydia. The former causes a very severe infection which becomes apparent two to four days after birth. It quickly involves the corneae and the resulting corneal ulcers may perforate rapidly with loss of the eyes. Chlamydial infection occurs later and is less serious.

Management. As soon as the condition is suspected the baby's eyes should be examined and cultures prepared. Care must be taken not to damage the corneae during examination and the examiner should avoid pus spurting into his own eyes. Treatment is started with intensive local antibiotics (one drop every minute for five minutes, then one drop every five minutes for one hour, then hourly) until the discharge lessens. Penicillin drops are the treatment of choice in gonococcal infection. These drops should be freshly prepared. Chloramphenicol drops may be given while the pharmacist prepares the penicillin solution. Systemic penicillin should also be given in cases of gonococcal infection. Tetracyline drops are suitable for chlamydial infection. Treatment may need to be modified when the results of bacterial culture become known. The infant should be barrier nursed.

Viral and Chlamydial Conjunctivitis

This is usually relatively mild and it may be unilateral. Such conjunctivitis may be associated with fever, a sore throat and enlargement of the lymph glands. Discharge is scanty and mucoid. Punctate keratitis is a frequent accompaniment (chapter 13). Chlamydia are sensitive to tetracycline and sulphonamide drops. There is no specific treatment for virus conjunctivitis but it is usual to give chloramphenicol drops to prevent secondary bacterial infection. Chlamydial and viral conjunctivitis may persist for many months and steroid drops are sometimes given in such refractory cases for they relieve symptoms. However, they must never be given without close ophthalmic supervision in view of the complications that they can cause.

Acute Allergic Conjunctivitis

Susceptible children may develop an acute allergic reaction to certain grass pollens or some animals. The conjunctiva becomes oedematous and there is intense itching. The jelly-like swelling of the conjunctiva (chemosis) looks alarming but quickly subsides. Antihistamine drops (Otrivine-Antistin) may speed recovery.

Spring Catarrh (Vernal Catarrh)

This is a chronic allergic conjunctivitis. Sufferers may have other allergic conditions, for example, hay fever or asthma. Patients' symptoms are worse in the spring and summer. The eyes are sore, itchy and watery. Patients rub their eyes frequently and they may dislodge strands of mucus. The conjunctiva is red and irregularly thickened. Eversion of the upper lid may reveal a plaque of 'Cobblestone' papillae (Figure 12.1). White nodules may be present at the limbus (Figure 12.2). Occasionally corneal ulcers develop.

Treatment with sodium chromoglycate drops (Opticrom) is usually sufficient to control symptoms in milder cases. Severe cases need local steroids which, again, should only be given under close ophthalmic supervision.

Figure 12.1: Cobblestone Papillae

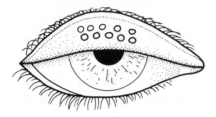

Figure 12.2 Cornea in Vernal Catarrh

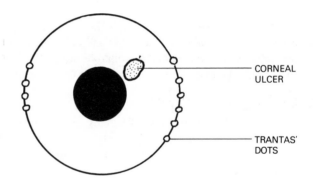

CORNEAL
ULCER

TRANTAS'
DOTS

Trachoma

This is an infection of the conjunctiva with *Chlamydia trachomatis*. Patients
tend to have recurrent attacks resulting in chronic disease of the conjunctiva and
cornea. It is one of the commonest causes of blindness in the Middle East and it
may be seen in immigrants to the United Kingdom. The disease may be spread
by flies which carry infected conjunctival secretions from person to person.

Symptoms and Signs

At first the attacks resemble an acute viral conjunctivitis. Later, blood vessels
pass into the upper part of the cornea and corneal opacities develop (Figure
12.3).

After several attacks the conjunctiva becomes scarred. It shrinks, so causing
entropion of both the upper and lower lids. The eye is dry as conjunctival secretions are reduced. Progressive corneal scarring develops due to the in-turned
lashes constantly abrading the cornea. These dry eyes are particularly prone to
secondary infection which further contributes to the corneal scarring.

Figure 12.3: Pannus

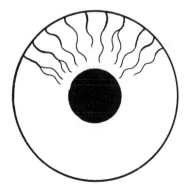

Treatment

The acute inflammation is treated with local or systemic tetracycline or sulphonamides. Chronic cases may require surgery to correct both entropion and trichiasis (chapter 10).

Prevention of Blindness Due to Trachoma

This depends upon early and thorough treatment of acute attacks and any lid complications. The regular washing of hands and faces and the reduction of the fly population helps to reduce the spread of the disease.

Pemphigus

This is a condition of unknown cause associated with blistering of the skin and mild conjunctivitis.

Benign Mucus Membrane Pemphigoid

Again, the cause of this condition is unknown. It is associated with progressive inflammation, ulceration and shrinkage of the conjunctiva. Blindness may result.

Conjunctival Degenerations

These affect particularly those parts of the conjunctiva that are exposed to the elements when the eye is open. Pinqueculae are harmless fatty plaques which may be excised if they are very unsightly. A pterygium is a wing-shaped mass of thickened conjunctiva which grows on to the cornea. It should be excised before it encroaches upon the central part of the cornea. This may be done under local anaesthesia. The area of bare sclera is left to re-epithelialise from the adjacent cornea and conjunctiva. Unfortunately, recurrence is relatively common and further excision of the pterygium, closely followed by β-irradiation, may be necessary to effect a cure.

Conjunctival Pigmentation

The long-term use of adrenaline drops (Eppy, Simplene, etc.) may cause tiny black deposits to form in the conjunctiva. These are quite harmless but they may be mistaken for foreign bodies.

Conjunctival Tumours

These are rare. Melanomas may be benign or malignant. The former are small pigmented lesions which should be left alone. Any increase in pigmentation or vascularity suggests that malignant change has occurred and the tumour should be widely excised.

Bowen's disease is a carcinoma which has not yet invaded the surrounding tissues. It should be completely excised. Squamous carcinoma and malignant melanoma may be so advanced by the time the patient presents that enucleation or exenteration may be required in order to achieve complete removal of the tumour.

13 DISEASES OF THE CORNEA

Patients who develop corneal problems usually seek advice promptly. This is because most corneal disorders reduce the transparency of the cornea and this results in the vision becoming blurred.

Congenital and Hereditary Diseases of the Cornea

Keratoconus

In this condition the cornea becomes progressively more conical with thinning and weakening (ectasia) of its central portion (Figure 13.1). It characteristically develops in early adult life.

Figure 13.1: Keratoconus

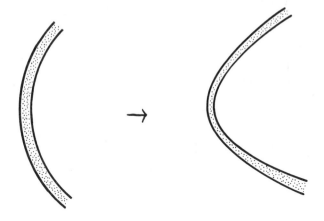

At first the patient complains of blurred vision because the light rays are refracted unevenly by the distorted cornea. Initially, spectacles may correct this. Later a contact lens may enable the patient to see adequately but in advanced cases corneal grafting may be necessary. There may be episodes of 'acute hydrops' when Descemet's membrane ruptures at the apex of the cone, allowing aqueous to enter the stroma, thus causing corneal oedema. The irregularity of the corneal surface causes pain. The oedema leads to marked impairment of vision. This condition usually subsides spontaneously. Perforation of the cornea occurs only rarely.

Keratoconus may be detected by observing the conical shape of the cornea with a slit-lamp microscope. Alternatively, the distortion of the corneal surface may be identified using a Placido's disc. The reflections on the cornea of the concentric circles on the disc are viewed through a central aperture. Distorted reflections betray the irregular corneal surface. If the cornea is markedly conical then the lower lid may take up an equivalent configuration when the patient looks downwards.

Corneal Dystrophies

These are uncommon hereditary conditions which usually become apparent in adolescence. Tiny opacities develop in the cornea which gradually increase in size. They often impair vision. Some types of dystrophy involve the epithelium causing multiple tiny painful ulcers. Corneal grafting may improve the patient's vision but the dystrophy often recurs in the graft.

Corneal Degenerations

Arcus Senilis

This is a narrow white band which appears in the peripheral cornea of the elderly (Figure 13.2.) It does not impair vision. A similar condition appearing in young people may be a sign of abnormal serum lipids.

Figure 13.2: Arcus Senilis

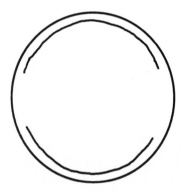

Band Degeneration

This is a white plaque which appears in the lower half of the cornea, at first peripherally and later centrally (Figure 13.3). If often occurs in eyes which have poor vision as a consequence of iritis or glaucoma. Occasionally it occurs in otherwise normal eyes, in which case the patient's vision may be improved by chemically removing the calcium salts by dissolving them with disodium versonate. (This may be done in the Out-patient Department.)

Figure 13.3: Band Degeneration

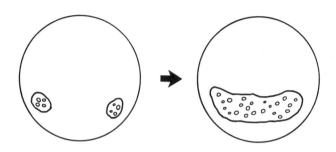

Fuchs's Dystrophy and Cornea Guttata

The corneal endothelium is responsible for pumping water out of the cornea, thus keeping it transparent (see chapter 2). In Fuchs's Dystrophy this 'endothelial pump' fails and the cornea becomes oedematous. The resultant blurring of vision is particularly marked in the mornings. Elderly people are those most commonly affected. They have often had guttata for many years. (Guttata are brown spots seen on the endothelium with the slit-lamp microscope.)

Patients with cornea guttata and Fuchs's Dystrophy are particularly likely to develop bullous keratopathy after cataract surgery. This is because the necessary manipulation of the cornea entailed during the operation further damages the endothelium.

Bullous Keratopathy

This is a condition in which the cornea is so oedematous that blisters (bullae) appear on its surface. Not only is the vision blurred but the eye is painful because corneal nerve endings are exposed when the bullae burst. The keratopathy is due to the endothelial pump failing. It may follow intraocular operations or be the end result of diseases such as *Herpes simplex* keratitis or Fuchs's Dystrophy.

A corneal graft (with healthy donor endothelium) is occasionally successful in relieving both the pain and the visual loss. If the patient is not suitable for grafting his pain may be relieved by his wearing a soft contact lens.

Inflammatory Disease of the Cornea. Keratitis and Corneal Ulcers

Keratitis means inflammation of the cornea. It is a potentially serious condition which may eventually result in blindness. It may be due to injury, surgery, infection or a variety of mechanical and nutritional factors. Corneal infections are sometimes secondary to conjunctivitis or dacryocystitis.

Signs and Symptoms

Keratitis may involve the whole cornea or be confined to a small area of it. It may involve the whole thickness of the cornea or be limited to either its superficial or deep layers. When only the epithelium is inflamed, its cells die and slough, leaving an area that stains green with fluorescein; this is a superficial corneal ulcer. When only the deeper layers are involved (deep keratitis) there is no ulcer but a grey or white area where the cornea is swollen and opaque; this is because inflammation interferes with the metabolic processes which normally keep the cornea transparent (see chapter 2). When both the epithelium and the deeper layers are involved there is a deep corneal ulcer with a white base and a central area which stains green with fluorescein (Figure 13.4).

Figure 13.4: Superficial Corneal Ulcer; Deep Keratitis; Deep Corneal Ulcer

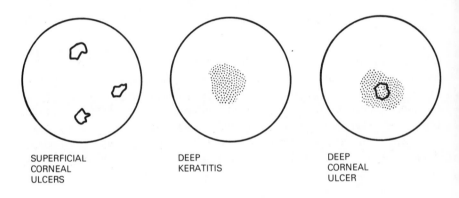

SUPERFICIAL   DEEP   DEEP
CORNEAL   KERATITIS   CORNEAL
ULCERS   ULCER

Corneal ulcers are painful because the corneal nerve endings lose their protective covering of epithelium. There is often considerable photophobia and lacrimation. There is usually some degree of iritis and in severe cases there may be an hypopyon.

Course and Complications

Most forms of keratitis are slow to heal and are followed by scarring which may permanently impair vision. Healing may be speeded up by blood vessels growing from the limbus into the patch of keratitis, bringing phagocytes and antibodies with them. However, such vascularisation is undesirable because it adds to the loss of transparency and may cause any corneal graft to become opaque.

Some corneal ulcers appear loath to heal and are termed indolent. Others spread rapidly to involve a larger area and deeper layers. If the ulcer becomes so deep that only Descemet's membrane is left, the membrane bulges under the influence of the intraocular pressure as a descemetocele (Figure 13.5). The slightest trauma may cause a descemetocele to perforate. Aqueous then escapes unless the perforation is sealed by a knuckle of iris.

Although perforation may be followed by healing, the eye is usually considerably disorganised. The iris may adhere to the cornea forming an anterior synechia. The term 'leucoma adherens' is used to describe such a synechia associated with a dense corneal scar. A cataract may develop and glaucoma may ensue.

Investigation

The cause of keratitis can often be determined by examining the patient either with the naked eye or, preferably, with a slit-lamp microscope. To determine the nature of any infective organisms, it is necessary to send conjunctival swabs and perhaps corneal scrapings to the microbiology laboratory for analysis.

Treatment

The general aims of treatment are to combat infection, reduce inflammation, treat iritis, promote healing and relieve pain.

Treatment of Infection

Corneal ulcers which are primarily due to infection should be treated with intensive antibiotic, anti-viral or anti-fungal drugs. Antibiotics are also given to those patients with ulcers due to nutritional or mechanical causes in the hope of preventing secondary infection. Carbolisation (or iodisation) is a useful procedure to cure dendritic ulcers (see below). This approach is particularly useful when anti-viral therapy is either contra-indicated (e.g., in pregnancy), or when it has been unsuccessful.

Carbolisation (Iodisation). This procedure is usually carried out in the Outpatients' Department. The affected eye is anaesthetised with cocaine and a lid retractor is inserted. It may be necessary to instil fluorescein and to use a microscope to delineate the ulcer precisely. The eye is dried with sterile filter paper. Carbolic acid (or iodine in an alcoholic solution) is applied to the base and edges of the ulcer on the tip of of an orange stick. The orange stick should be kept well clear of the conjunctiva. After iodisation, further cocaine is instilled in order to fix the iodine. Once treated, the corneal epithelium becomes white. Finally, an antibiotic ointment and a pad and bandage are applied. The patient should be warned that the eye will be painful for a few hours; he should go home to bed and take oral analgesics as required. The ulcer may appear larger the next day because the treated epithelium sloughs, but 48 hours later healing should be well advanced.

Reduction of Inflammation

Steroid drops are sometimes given, once the infection is brought under control, so as to reduce inflammation more rapidly, thus minimising corneal scarring.

Figure 13.5: Descemetocele and Anterior Synechia

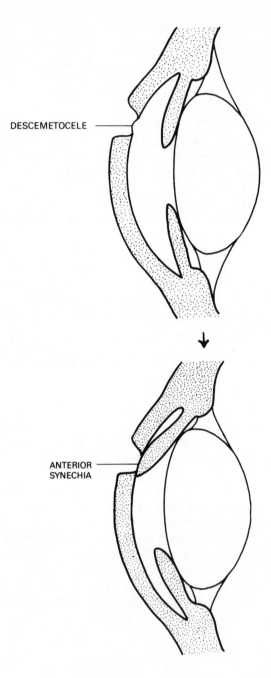

However, this should only be done under close supervision because the infection may break out again and the epithelium fail to heal. This warning applies part-icularly to *Herpes simplex* keratitis.

Treatment of Iritis

Mydriatics should be given both to break down posterior synechiae and also to relieve pain by reducing ciliary spasm. Steroids may be given if it is considered safe to do so.

Promotion of Healing

A corneal ulcer is more likely to heal if the eye is kept closed, as this avoids repeated damage to the epithelium by movements of the lids. In the case of a simple ulcer, closing the eye with a pad and bandage is sufficient. It is important that the lids do not open under the pad, or the pad itself may abrade the cornea. A pad should not be used when there is conjunctivitis, as it will retain infected secretions.

Those ulcers due to exposure or impaired sensation of the cornea may not heal until the lids have been sewn together. A tarsorrhaphy is a relatively minor operation which can be performed under local anaesthesia (e.g., amethocaine drops and lid infiltration with lignocaine). The epithelium of the conjunctival half of the lid margin is excised and the lids stitched together over lengths of tubing (Figure 13.6).

Either the central or the lateral parts of the lids can be united depending upon the extent of closure of the eye that is judged appropriate (Figure 13.7).

Figure 13.6: Tarsorrhaphy — Method

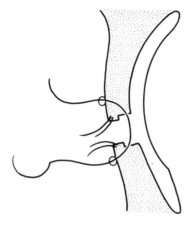

Figure 13.7: Tarsorrhaphy — Types

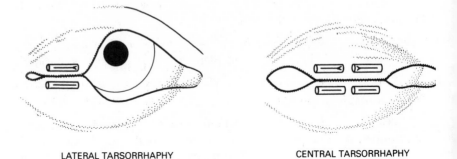

LATERAL TARSORRHAPHY   CENTRAL TARSORRHAPHY

Special Features

Herpes Simplex Keratitis

Herpex simplex is the virus that causes the 'cold sores' around the nose and mouth which afflict most people from time to time. It is also one of the commonest causes of keratitis in the United Kingdom. It often starts as a dendritic ulcer. This is a superficial corneal ulcer with a typical branching appearance (Figure 13.8). It can often be seen with the naked eye after fluorescein has been instilled. Initially, it may be treated by carbolisation (or iodisation) or by the anti-viral agent idoxuridine (IDU). IDU is best given as ointment five times daily for at least ten days. If one method fails, the other may be tried. Vidarabine (Vira-A), trifluorothymidine (F_3T) and acyclovir (Zovirax) are newer anti-virals which may be prescribed for such cases.

Figure 13.8: Dendritic Ulcer

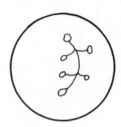

It is very dangerous to give steroid drops for a dendritic ulcer. The ulcer gets rapidly worse and it takes longer to heal. However, if steroids have been given (i.e., before the diagnosis was made) they must be withdrawn only slowly for otherwise, paradoxically, the ulcer may get worse.

Herpes simplex may also cause deep corneal ulcers, usually in patients who have had dendritic ulcers in the past. Another common sequel is disciform keratitis — a round patch of deep keratitis usually affecting the central cornea. Disciform keratitis clears more rapidly if steroid drops are given but they should be used only in conjunction with anti-viral therapy and only under close supervision.

Superficial Punctate Keratitis

Some viruses (e.g., *Adenovirus, Herpes simplex*) and *Chlamydiae* (e.g., *Tric agent*) may cause a superficial keratitis. The cornea is covered with multiple tiny ulcers which can be seen only with the slit-lamp microscope (Figure 13.9).

Figure 13.9: Superficial Punctate Keratitis

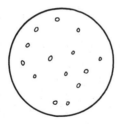

The condition subsides spontaneously after several days or weeks; a few cases are left with punctate scars. There is no specific treatment for adenovirus infection; usually antibiotics (e.g., chloramphenicol drops) are given to prevent secondary infection. Steroid drops ease the discomfort and may be given if *Herpes simplex* keratitis can be excluded. Chlamydiae are sensitive to tetracycline, which can be given orally, or as drops or ointment.

Herpes Zoster Ophthalmicus ('Shingles')

The *Herpes zoster* virus causes chickenpox in children and young adults. After this infection, the virus lies dormant in nerves and may cause an outbreak of 'shingles' in later life. Characteristically, the 'shingles' rash is limited to the skin supplied by one or two cutaneous nerves on one side of the body.

Herpes zoster ophthalmicus means 'shingles' affecting the first (ophthalmic) division of the trigeminal nerve and the structures supplied by it. These are the skin of the forehead and scalp, the nose and the upper lid and the conjunctiva and the globe. Often the eye itself is spared, particularly, so some say, if the nose is free of vesicles. Occasionally, *Herpes zoster* is the first sign that the patient's immune responses are impaired by a disease such as leukaemia. Thus a thorough medical examination should be carried out.

Symptoms and Signs. Initially pain develops in the forehead and in the eye. After a few days, vesicles appear which become progessively larger and then burst before forming crusts. Finally, the scabs drop off to leave depressed scars. The eye may be affected in several ways. Conjunctivitis and small corneal ulcers are common. More serious complications include corneal anaesthesia (see p.116), iritis, secondary glaucoma and a paralytic squint. All these signs may initially be hidden by the marked swelling of the upper lid which often prevents the patient opening the eye.

Treatment. All patients with *Herpes zoster* ophthalmicus should be seen by an ophthalmologist who should examine the eye carefully and advise on treatment. Admission to hospital may be required if the patient has no one to nurse him at home. He is infectious until the last scab has dropped off and so isolation in a single room is necessary. Strong analgesics may be required to control pain. The skin may be treated with a combined antibiotic and steroid ointment or with an idoxuridine preparation such as 'Herpid' or with acyclovir ointment. Once the vesicles start to burst and form crusts, then regular skin toilet is necessary. Steroid drops and mydriatics are given for iritis and acetazolamide for glaucoma. A tarsorrhaphy may be necessary to protect an anaesthetic cornea once the eye opens. The patient may continue to be afflicted by pain (post-herpetic neuralgia) and by many of the ocular complications even after the skin has cleared so that long-term follow-up may be necessary.

Bacterial Keratitis

This usually follows trauma to the cornea, e.g., corneal abrasion or removal of a foreign body. Pneumococci or Pseudomonas are usually responsible. It is often a very serious condition with a large necrotic ulcer and an hypopyon. The ulcer may rapidly deepen and lead to the eye perforating.

The patient should be admitted to hospital and given intensive antibiotic treatment (e.g., hourly drops by day and ointment at night with sub-conjunctival injections and systemic antibiotics in severe cases). Occasionally a paracentesis of the anterior chamber is performed; this releases pus which may be sent for culture. If the infection progresses to fill the whole globe (panophthalmitis) there is almost no hope of preserving sight and it is best to perform an evisceration (chapter 24). Keratitis may also be caused by the *Gonococcus* (chapter 12).

Marginal Ulcers

Bacterial conjunctivitis is sometimes accompanied by corneal ulcers which can be seen as white spots at the periphery of the cornea (Figure 13.10). The causative organism is usually *Staphylococcus aureus*. These ulcers will heal provided the conjunctivitis is treated with appropriate antibiotic drugs. Any resulting scars do not affect the patient's vision, for the central part of the cornea is not involved.

Figure 13.10: Marginal Ulcers

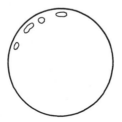

Interstitial Keratitis

This is a form of deep keratitis which occurs in children and young adults with congenital syphilis. It is uncommon nowadays. The keratitis is bilateral and painful and causes corneal scarring with vascularisation. Steroids and mydriatics are given locally and Penicillin is given systemically. The cornea clears over a period of months or years and the patient's vision may eventually be quite good.

Fungal Keratitis

A fungus infection is characteristically acquired when the cornea is injured in gardening or farming accidents. The ulcer is usually indolent with an associated hypopyon. Fungus infection may be superimposed upon a primary viral or bacterial corneal infection particularly if local immunity has been suppressed by steroid drops. Only a few antifungal agents are suitable for ophthalmic use and treatment is not always successful.

Keratitis due to Nutritional Factors

Vitamin A Deficiency

This is a common cause of blindness in developing countries. The conjunctiva becomes dry due to lack of secretions (xerophthalmia). The cornea becomes dry and insensitive and then simply melts away. Immediate treatment with large doses of vitamin A may save such eyes. Night blindness (due to lack of vitamin A in the retina) develops before xerophthalmia becomes apparent.

Acne Rosacea

This may affect the eyes in addition to causing a red pimply rash on the face.

Ulcers develop at the edge of the cornea; they heal leaving faceted and vascularised scars. Treatment with steroid drops is often beneficial.

Mooren's Ulcer

This is a painful indolent ulcer at the edge of the cornea. It occurs in old people. There is no specific treatment.

Keratitis due to Mechanical Factors

Keratitis is prone to develop whenever the normal protective mechanisms of the eye are impaired (chapter 2). Secondary infection is likely to follow and cause further damage to the eye.

Neurotrophic Keratitis (Anaesthetic Cornea)

This may be due to injuries, infections (e.g., *Herpes zoster*) or operations which damage the trigeminal nerve (V_1). The patient does not experience pain when the cornea is damaged. Corneal foreign bodies or infections may initially go undetected by the patient. Extensive ulceration of the cornea may be present by the time the patient seeks advice.

Treatment includes the regular instillation of antibiotic drops to prevent infection. The lids should be kept closed at night by securing a pad over the closed lids with adhesive tape. A tarsorrhaphy may be advisable.

Keratoconjunctivitis Sicca (Dry Eye)

Dryness of the eyes is commonly complicated by corneal ulceration (chapter 11). Treatment consists of improving the lubrication of the eyes and routine treatment of any ulcer that may arise.

Neuroparalytic Keratitis (Defective Lid Closure)

If the eyelids do not close properly, the cornea is likely to become dry and ulcerated. Inefficient blinking adds to the problem, for any tears that are present are not evenly distributed over the cornea. Inadequate closure of the lids may be due to lesions of the facial nerve and occurs in Bell's palsy, cerebrovascular accidents, following the removal of an acoustic neuroma, scarring of the eyelids from burns or lacerations, thyrotoxicosis and in those patients who are in coma.

It is often necessary to perform a tarsorrhaphy but in mild cases the liberal application of ointment at night may provide sufficient protection of the cornea.

Trichiasis

In-turned eyelashes (see 'Trichiasis', p.87) may cause chronic corneal ulceration. Treatment consists of electrolysis, cryotherapy, or lid surgery to deal with the offending lashes as well as routine treatment of any ulcers.

Corneal Grafting (Keratoplasty)

Because the cornea is avascular (and therefore not readily reached by circulating antibodies) corneal grafts are less likely to be rejected than are other organ grafts. Usually, only the central portion of the cornea is replaced so that the limbal blood vessels and the drainage angle are not damaged by the operation.

Indications

Corneal grafts are most often performed to improve the vision of those patients with corneal scarring (from keratitis or trauma), keratoconus or corneal dystrophies. Because of the inevitable risks of the operation, grafting is usually reserved for patients with an acuity of 6/36 or less. Those eyes that are dry or those with either anaesthetic or vascularised corneas, are often judged unsuitable for grafting.

Occasionally grafting is performed as an emergency for a perforated corneal ulcer.

Collection of Donor Material

Donor eyes should be removed within six hours of the death of the donor. Graft material is usually obtained from the bodies of those who, during their lifetime, gave written consent to their eyes being removed after their death. Sometimes the next of kin may ask that their dead relative's eyes be used to restore a patient's eyesight. If the relatives cannot be contacted then the coroner may allow the eyes to be removed. Occasionally the cornea of an eye that has been enucleated because of the presence of a choroidal melanoma may be used for grafting.

The eyes are usually removed by a junior surgeon who goes to the house or hospital where the donor died. He should take with him a pack of sterile equipment which has been kept in readiness at the Eye Hospital. He takes conjunctival swabs from the donor and irrigates the eyes with antibiotic solutions. He then removes the eyes, using a sterile technique (chapter 24), and places them in dry sterile containers.

On returning to the Eye Hospital the surgeon should send the conjunctival swabs to the Microbiology Department. The eyes are either kept at 4°C, and used within 24 hours, or sent to the nearest Eye Bank. At the Eye Bank, the cornea, with a rim of sclera, is dissected from the eye. It may then be kept in McCarey-Kaufman medium at 4°C, and used within four to seven days, or frozen in liquid nitrogen at −196°C and kept even longer.

Types of Graft

Penetrating keratoplasty involves replacing all the corneal layers with the donor corneal disc. Usually a central disc of the patient's cornea measuring 7 or 8 millimetres in diameter is replaced (Figure 13.11). Smaller grafts tend to give poor visual results and larger ones may damage the drainage angle, causing glaucoma.

Lamellar keratoplasty entails replacing a disc of partial thickness leaving Descemet's membrane and the endothelium intact. Because the anterior chamber is not entered, the operative risks are reduced; a bigger disc may be replaced. However, some degree of scarring always occurs between the graft and the recipient cornea so that the visual results are often disappointing (Figure 13.12). Of course, lamellar keratoplasty is inappropriate when the corneal scarring involves the deeper layers of the stroma or where the recipient endothelium is diseased.

Figure 13.11: Penetrating Keratoplasty

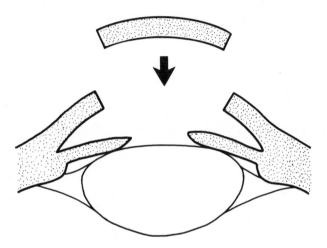

Figure 13.12: Lamellar Keratoplasty

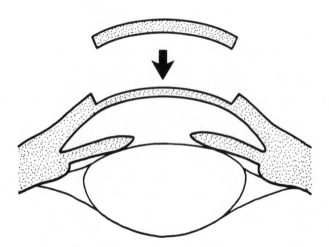

Method of Penetrating Keratoplasty

This operation is best carried out under general anaesthesia. Pre-operatively, the pupil is constricted with pilocarpine drops so that if the trephine enters the eye too deeply, then the iris is engaged rather than the anterior lens capsule. The intraocular pressure is lowered with intravenous mannitol or Diamox. Antibiotic drops are instilled. The eye is immobilised with fixation sutures in the superior and inferior recti and it is then covered with moistened gauze while the donor material is prepared.

The donor eye is dipped in an antibiotic solution and a piece of gauze is wrapped around it so that it may be held firmly. Some surgeons rub off the epithelium because it contains antigens. A corneal disc of suitable size is cut with the trephine. Sometimes, both eyes of the pair are trephined and the better disc is selected. The corneal disc is placed, epithelium downwards, on a watch glass while the recipient's eye is trephined using the same instrument. On the donor eye the trephining may be swift and relatively forceful as damage to the intraocular structures is irrelevant. However, on the recipient's eye trephining has to be slow and careful and once aqueous escapes, removal of the disc should be completed with curved scissors or a blade. (If a corneo-scleral disc from the Eye Bank is used, the disc is placed epithelium downwards and the trephining done from the endothelial side.)

The diseased corneal disc is then removed and replaced with the donor disc. Handling of the donor disc is kept to a minimum to reduce damage to the endothelium. The excised disc of the patient's cornea is sent for histological examination.

Suturing is best carried out under the operating microscope with 10/0 monofilament nylon. Either continuous or interrupted sutures may be used (Figure 13.13). In the former case, four interrupted silk sutures are inserted initially to stabilise the graft; they may be removed at the end of the operation. Sufficient sutures are inserted to make the eye watertight and the anterior chamber is re-formed with saline. Antibiotic drops are instilled and the eye is closed with a pad and bandage.

Figure 13.13: Corneal Graft — Suturing

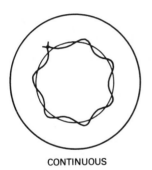 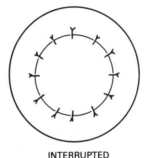

CONTINUOUS   INTERRUPTED

After-care

The eye is usually inspected at either 24 or 48 hours post-operatively as complications may require re-operation at this early stage. Antibiotics, steroids and mydriatics are instilled according to the surgeon's preference. The patient is then mobilised. If the eye is healing well then dark glasses may be worn by day but the patient should continue to wear a pad at night.

The patient is discharged from hospital about a week after the operation. He continues using steroid drops at home and is closely supervised in the Outpatient Clinic. Nylon sutures are left in the eye for several months, or indefinitely if they become covered by epithelium. A refraction may be performed and suitable lenses prescribed after about six weeks but several changes of lenses may be necessary during the subsequent year or two whilst the eye gradually heals.

Complications of Grafting

As with any intraocular operation infection, haemorrhage and sympathetic ophthalmia may occur.

Flat Anterior Chamber. If the wound is not watertight, aqueous will escape and the anterior chamber becomes flat. This is usually noted at the first dressing. Occasionally, firm bandaging alone will allow healing and reformation of the anterior chamber to occur but resuturing in theatre may be necessary.

Iris Prolapse. This may be due to leakage of the wound or to pupil block glaucoma, or to both these complications. Some surgeons perform peripheral iridectomies before suturing the graft in place in order to reduce the risk of pupil block. If it does occur, then the prolapsed iris should be replaced or be removed (abscised) and the wound resutured in theatre.

Tilting of the Graft. This will cause astigmatism which may necessitate the patient wearing a contact lens to correct it.

Opacification of the Graft. The graft may become opaque at any time for several reasons. In the first few weeks infection, glaucoma or a leaking wound may be the cause. After this the cause may be recurrence of the original disease (e.g., *Herpes simplex*) or an ageing endothelium (see 'Fuchs's Dystrophy', p.107) or graft rejection.

Graft Rejection. Corneal graft rejection does occur although it is much less common than rejection of other grafts (e.g., kidney). It is most likely to happen if the graft becomes vascularised. If it is recognised in time and intensive local steroids given, the graft may become clear again.

Keratoprosthesis

A disc of acrylic may be used to replace a scarred cornea instead of using a corneal graft. Insertion of a keratoprosthesis is technically difficult and post-operative complications are common so this technique is reserved for patients in whom corneal grafting has failed.

14 SCLERA

The sclera is the tough white outer coat of the eye.

Congenital Disorders

In osteogenesis imperfecta (fragilatas ossium) the sclera is thin and appears blue. This of itself usually causes no problems. However, should squint surgery be undertaken the surgeon must take extreme care in placing sutures in the sclera.

Episcleritis

This is an inflammation of the episcleral tissues, which lie between the sclera and the conjunctiva. The patient complains of discomfort and of a red patch on the eye. Episcleritis does not threaten sight and it resolves spontaneously. Local steroids may be used to shorten the period of discomfort.

Scleritis

This is a much more serious disorder in which the sclera itself is inflamed; the overlying episclera and conjunctiva may also become involved. The entire sclera may be inflamed or only part of it be affected. It may complicate general disorders such as rheumatoid arthritis.

In anterior scleritis the patient complains of severe pain. The eye is red and there may be a nodule in the sclera. In posterior uveitis the patient's vision may be blurred because a serous retinal detachment may develop.

Treatment is with systemic steroids. The sclera may be permanently thinned and weakened after such an attack. A staphyloma (bulging of the sclera and underlying choroid) may develop and occasionally the eye perforates (scleromalacia perforans).

15 THE UVEA

The uvea or uveal tract is composed of the iris, ciliary body and choroid.

Congenital Anomalies

Abnormal development may result in iris anomalies such as a keyhole-shaped defect in the iris (coloboma) or an eccentric pupil (corectopia) (Figure 15.1). The vision may be poor, not because of the iris defect but because of an associated retinal lesion.

Figure 15.1: Iris Anomalies

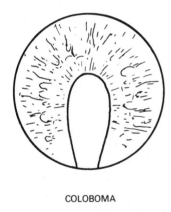

COLOBOMA

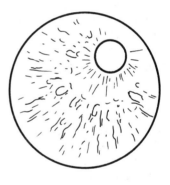

CORECTOPIA

Inflammation

Inflammation of the uvea, or uveitis, is a relatively common ophthalmic problem. It may threaten the eyesight in many ways. The inflammation is usually predominantly either anterior or posterior, although occasionally the entire uvea is affected — a pan-uveitis. In anterior uveitis the iris and the ciliary body are inflamed and so it may be called iritis or iridocyclitis. In posterior uveitis the choroid is inflamed; usually the adjacent retina is also affected so it may be called choroiditis or retino-choroiditis.

Anterior Uveitis (Iritis, Iridocyclitis)

Cause

Iritis may occur in association with diseases such as ankylosing spondylitis, sarcoidosis, tuberculosis or syphilis. Some degree of iritis occurs after intraocular operations, after ocular trauma and in association with corneal ulcers. Very often, however, no cause can be found. Sympathetic ophthalmia and heterochromic cyclitis have special features and are considered separately.

Symptoms

Iritis commonly has an acute onset. The patient attends the Casualty Department with a painful red eye. The pain may be quite severe and disturb sleep. The pain is due partly to spasm of the ciliary muscle. The redness is often most marked around the cornea ('ciliary' or 'circumcorneal' injection). The vision may be slightly blurred and there may be some photophobia and watering of the eye. Sometimes the second eye becomes affected a few days later. Occasionally the iritis has a more insidious onset. The patient notices blurred vision but there is not much pain or redness of the eye.

Signs

Many of the signs of iritis are only visible with the slit-lamp microscope. With this instrument white cells can be seen circulating in the aqueous; they look like the dust particles seen in the beam of light from a slide projector. The aqueous contains protein which has exuded from the blood vessels of the inflamed iris and ciliary body. The high protein content of the aqueous causes the slit-lamp beam to appear white as it crosses the anterior chamber causing a 'flare'. This is akin to the beam of light from an usherette's torch showing up in a smoky cinema. (Normally when the slit-lamp beam is shone across the anterior chamber no cells can be seen and the beam of light is transparent.) Sometimes so much protein is exuded that it collects in a mass which may occlude the pupil.

The inflamed iris becomes sticky and adhesions may form between the pupil margin and the lens. These adhesions are called posterior synechiae. Initially they are difficult to detect but when a mydriatic is instilled they become obvious because the pupil dilates irregularly (Figure 15.2).

If the entire pupillary margin adheres to the lens no aqueous can pass from the posterior to the anterior chamber. Aqueous then rapidly builds up behind the iris and pushes it forward (iris bombé), while the intraocular pressure rises (Figure 15.3).

Inflammatory cells are deposited on the back of the cornea as keratic precipitates. Sometimes they are big enough to see with the naked eye and look greasy, like globules of mutton fat.

In severe cases, sufficient inflammatory cells are shed to form an hypopyon — a collection of pus in the anterior chamber (Figure 15.4).

Figure 15.2: Posterior Synechiae

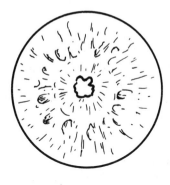

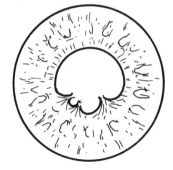

BEFORE MYDRIATIC   AFTER MYDRIATIC

Figure 15.3: Iris Bombé

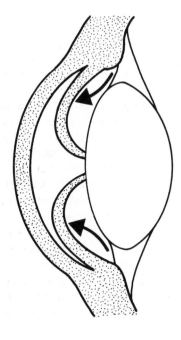

Figure 15.4: Hypopyon

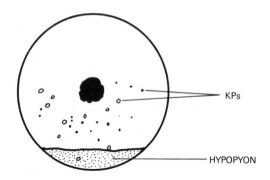

Granulomatous Iritis

This is the name given to those cases which show mutton fat keratic precipitates, nodules in the iris and granulomata on histological examination. It is often found to be due to sarcoidosis and tends to have a more chronic course. Non-granulomatous iritis, with smaller keratic precipitates and without nodules and granulomata, is more common.

With correct treatment iritis tends to subside within a few weeks. The signs and symptoms may disappear completely but often pigmented keratic precipitates, posterior synechiae and pigmented deposits on the lens remain as evidence of the attack. However, further attacks frequently occur after intervals of weeks, months or years. Some cases never completely subside but grumble on for years as a chronic condition; these cases are particularly likely to develop complications.

Complications

Secondary Glaucoma. A rise in the intraocular pressure may be due either to iris bombé or to the blockage of the aqueous drainage channels by inflammatory cells and exudate.

Secondary Cataract. Lens opacities may develop because the nutrition of the lens is impaired while the eye is inflamed.

Band Keratopathy. Calcium salts may be deposited in the cornea if the inflammation is prolonged or recurrent (see chapter 13).

Phthisis Bulbi. In advanced cases the ciliary body may be so damaged that it fails to secrete aqueous. The intraocular pressure then falls and the eye shrinks into a sightless and scarred (but painless) remnant.

Investigations

It is usual to screen a patient with iritis for treatable diseases such as tuberculosis and syphilis by performing a blood count, ESR, chest X-ray and serum VDRL. More detailed investigation is usually not worthwhile.

Treatment

The aims of treatment are to control inflammation, to break down posterior synechiae, to relieve pain and treat any complications.

Control of Inflammation. Since the cause of the inflammation is usually unknown, all that can be done is to suppress it with anti-inflammatory drugs. (The rare infective causes such as syphilis require appropriate systemic antibiotics.) Treatment is usually started with steroid drops such as prednisolone (Predsol), betamethasone (Betnesol) or dexamethasone (Maxidex) given at one or two hourly intervals; later the frequency of instillation can be reduced.

Steroids can also be given subconjunctivally as a betamethasone or methylprednisolone (Depomedrone) injection. The latter preparation has a more prolonged effect but leaves an unsightly white deposit under the conjunctiva for several days which may cause conjunctival scarring. Subconjunctival injections are helpful when the iritis is severe or when patients are unwilling or unable to instil drops.

Occasionally, systemic steroids are necessary. They are usually given as prednisolone tablets. Systemic steroids may be dangerous in patients with tuberculosis and peptic ulceration so it is advisable to take a full medical history and a chest X-ray before prescribing them. Steroids may cause hypertension, diabetes mellitus and weight gain and so it is advisable to check frequently the patient's blood pressure, urine and weight. Patients who develop indigestion during treatment may be helped by taking the tablets with food or by taking enteric coated tablets, but sometimes treatment has to be stopped. Children on steroids may fail to grow, so treatment is usually given only in collaboration with a paediatrician.

Prevention and Treatment of Posterior Synechiae. Most cases of iritis tend to develop posterior synechiae with the risk of iris bombé and secondary glaucoma occurring. Mydriatics are given to dilate the pupil, thus breaking down posterior synechiae as the iris is pulled away from the lens. Ideally the patient should not leave the hospital until he has a round, dilated pupil and this may require many drops of strong mydriatics such as cyclopentolate, phenylephrine and atropine. Occasionally, a subconjunctival injection of mydricaine (which contains both atropine and adrenaline) is necessary. This preparation may cause tachycardia and can be dangerous in the elderly. Mydriatics should be continued until the iritis has nearly subsided; usually atropine drops are given two or three times daily. Lachesine may be substituted if the patient is allergic to atropine. Most mydriatics also cause cycloplegia; this is beneficial as it reduces some of the pain of iritis which is due to ciliary spasm. However, it may so impair the patient's vision that he is unable to work.

Relief of Pain. Usually the pain subsides once the steroid and mydriatic-cycloplegic drugs have taken effect. However, it may be necessary to give analgesics for one or two days and especially before a subconjunctival injection is given. Local heat is comforting. This may be provided in hospital by a Maddox heater or at home by a hot water bottle or by hot spoon bathing.

Treatment of Complications. The complications of iritis include raised intraocular pressure, cataract and phthisis.

   Raised Intraocular Pressure. (Provided it is not due to iris bombé.) This will eventually subside as the inflammation comes under control. In the meantime, acetazolamide (Diamox) may be given by mouth or intravenously if the pressure is very high.
   Iris bombé is occasionally relieved by intensive mydriatic therapy but usually an operation is necessary to make a hole in the iris through which aqueous can flow from the posterior to the anterior chamber. One approach is to perform a broad iridectomy (Figure 15.5). Pre-operatively acetazolamide and steroids are given to make the eye as quiet as possible. A laser iridotomy performed in the Out-patient Department may avoid the need for conventional surgery.

Figure 15.5: Broad Iridectomy for Iris Bombé

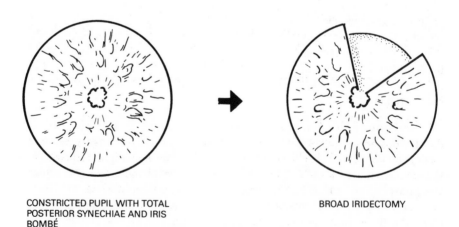

CONSTRICTED PUPIL WITH TOTAL
POSTERIOR SYNECHIAE AND IRIS
BOMBÉ

BROAD IRIDECTOMY

   Secondary Cataract. This may be removed once the eye has become reasonably quiet, but the operation is more hazardous than for a senile cataract and the visual results are often poor because of co-existing damage to the retina.

Phthisis Bulbi. No treatment will restore vision but the patient can wear a painted contact lens which may greatly improve his appearance.

Prognosis

Patients with iritis may lose their eyesight for many reasons, including corneal opacities, cataract and glaucoma. These complications are at least partly preventable by prompt and correct treatment. Because iritis may recur, patients should be warned to re-attend as soon as they have warning symptoms of iritis. It is also important to continue treatment until slit-lamp examination shows that the eye is completely quiet; this may be some time after the symptoms have disappeared.

Iritis and Ankylosing Spondylitis

Iritis occurs quite commonly in patients with ankylosing spondylitis. It is often severe, with an hypopyon. Because of the stiffness and deformity of the neck and back, patients may find it impossible to instil drops, so hospital admission and subconjunctival injections are often required.

Heterochromic Cyclitis

This is a form of chronic anterior uveitis in which the affected eye gradually loses iris pigment so that a brown eye becomes blue and a blue eye becomes paler. Usually just one eye is affected so that the two eyes become different in colour (heterochromia).

There is no pain or redness but cells, flare and keratic precipitates are seen with the slit-lamp. Synechiae characteristically do not develop, so that mydriatic drops are unnecessary. A cataract commonly develops; it can often be successfully removed, with a good visual result if the patient can wear a contact lens. A chronic glaucoma may develop so that the intraocular pressure should be checked regularly.

Sympathetic Ophthalmia

This is a bilateral granulomatous uveitis which follows a penetrating injury of one eye (see chapter 23). The inflammation starts in the injured eye and involves the second eye after a variable time interval (though virtually never earlier than ten days after the injury). The end result may be blindness in both eyes. To prevent this tragedy it is best to enucleate any eye which is persistently inflamed a week after a penetrating injury if it is blind or nearly so.

Posterior Uveitis (Choroiditis)

This is seen less often than anterior uveitis. It may be acute or chronic. The most common causes are toxoplasmosis and sarcoidosis.

Signs and Symptoms

The patient complains of blurred vision because the vitreous fills with inflammatory cells and exudates. He may complain of black blobs floating in his visual field. There is no pain unless the anterior uvea is also inflamed. On examination, viterous opacities can be seen with both the slit-lamp and the ophthalmoscope; they obsure the fundus view, sometimes completely. In toxoplasmosis the inflammation is confined to a single patch (or focus) of retina and choroid (chapter 19). In sarcoidosis the inflammation is more generalised.

Investigation

The underlying cause (toxoplasmosis, sarcoidosis) can often be determined from the appearance of the fundus, although this may not be visible until the vitreous opacities have cleared. It is usual to carry out screening tests such as a blood count and chest X-ray, but further investigations are often unnecessary.

Treatment

Systemic steroids are given to control the inflammation provided there is no medical contra-indication to their use. Local steroids and mydriatics are not required unless there is a co-existent iritis.

Prognosis

The patient's vision may return to normal once the acute attack has subsided, provided there was no focus of inflammation at the macula. However, if the choroiditis is chronic or recurrent, the vision tends to decline progressively due to vitreous opacification and retinal degeneration.

Toxocariasis

This is a uveal infection with the worm *Toxocara canis*, which infests most dogs. The worm is picked up by children who play in houses or parks frequented by dogs. It may cause a granuloma at the macula or a chronic pan-uveitis which leads to an endophthalmitis. A granuloma results in loss of central vision whilst an endophthalmitis causes total loss of sight in the affected eye.

Uveal Tumours

Benign Melanoma

This is a pigmented tumour which may be in the iris, ciliary body or choroid. Unlike a malignant melanoma it grows slowly, if at all. It is often detected only on routine examination.

Malignant Melanoma

This is a pigmented tumour which may arise in the iris, ciliary body or choroid — most commonly the latter. It may grow very rapidly and invade other ocular tissues. A choroidal melanoma tends to produce a serous retinal detachment so that the patient's vision worsens. Later, the vitreous is invaded, the globe fills with growth, the drainage angle is blocked and the eye becomes red, painful and blind due to glaucoma. Later, spread to the orbital tissues and eyelids may occur. Finally the tumour spreads to the liver with fatal results.

Investigations. It may be difficult to differentiate a small malignant melanoma of the choroid from a benign melanoma or a sub-choroidal haemorrhage. Sometimes the patient is observed for months or years and fundus photographs are taken regularly to see if the tumour is growing (and therefore probably malignant). A fluorescein angiogram and ultra-sonography may be helpful. Usually several consultant opinions are obtained if enucleation is contemplated.

Treatment. Very small malignant tumours may be treated by photocoagulation or radioactive cobalt plaques. Local excision may be appropriate but in many cases enucleation is necessary. Unfortunately, the tumour may already have metastasised and death from liver secondaries may still occur after enucleation.

Metastatic Carcinoma of the Choroid

Occasionally secondary tumours (metastases) occur in the choroid. The primary tumour is often in the breast. They may cause blurring of vision. They may be detected only on routine examination.

16 GLAUCOMA

Glaucoma is a condition in which the intraocular pressure is higher than the eye can tolerate and damage results. The way in which the eye suffers depends upon the degree of pressure elevation, its duration and the speed at which it develops.

Chronic Open-angle Glaucoma (Chronic Simple Glaucoma)

This is a relatively common disease of elderly people. In the United Kingdom the prevalence is about one in every hundred people over 40 years of age. It becomes progressively more common with increasing age. It tends to run in families.

Signs and Symptoms

There is no pain and externally the eye appears quite normal. The intraocular pressure is higher than normal and eventually may exceed 40mm Hg. The optic disc becomes increasingly pale and cupped (Figure 16.1).

Field defects appear, first para-centrally (Figure 16.2), then peripherally. In advanced cases the field is so constricted that there is 'tunnel vision'. The visual acuity may be normal until the last remnant of field is lost.

The disease usually affects one eye some time before the other but nearly always both eyes are eventually affected.

Complications

Branch and central retinal vein occlusions (chapter 19) commonly occur.

Presentation

Patients may be unaware that anything is wrong until they make a routine visit to their optician for spectacles. Opticians routinely inspect the optic discs and they may be the first to detect glaucomatous cupping. They may also have facilities for measuring the intraocular pressures and charting the visual fields.

Field defects are rarely noticed until they are quite advanced, in at least one eye. The sudden onset of blurred vision due to a venous occlusion may be the first warning of the disease.

Regular screening of persons with a family history of the disease allows early diagnosis, as does routine intraocular pressure measurement and scrutiny of the discs of all adults attending the Eye Department.

Figure 16.1: Disc Cupping (Left Eye)

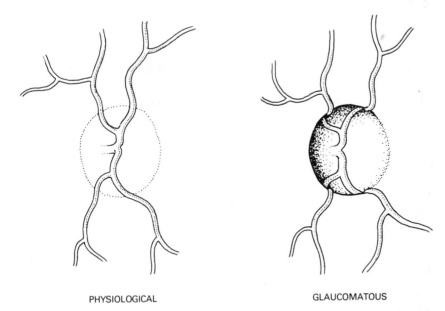

PHYSIOLOGICAL   GLAUCOMATOUS

Management

Once the diagnosis is made, the patient should be told that he has a condition that requires ophthalmic supervision for the rest of his life. He is seen frequently until his disease appears to be controlled by treatment. After this, four-monthly visits are usually sufficient. The visual acuity and intraocular pressures are measured and the discs are examined at every visit. The visual fields should be plotted every six to twelve months (chapter 5).

Initially, medical treatment is usually tried. Drugs are used either to increase the outflow of aqueous or decrease its production. Pilocarpine drops, in increasing concentration may be prescribed. Patients may give up these drops because they cause blurring of vision, especially in those young enough to have an appreciable power of accommodation (chapter 8). Neutral adrenaline is better tolerated in this connection, but it controls only mild cases. Timolol drops are often effective; acetazolamide by mouth may be used in resistant cases but it can have systemic side-effects. If necessary, a combination of drugs may be given; they usually have an additive effect.

When medical treatment is poorly tolerated or insufficient to control the intraocular pressure, or when field loss continues, either laser or conventional surgical treatment is advised. The aim of surgery is to increase the outflow of aqueous by providing an alternative drainage channel namely into the subconjunctival space (Figure 16.3). Scheie's operation is carried out by making an

Figure 16.2: Field Loss in Chronic Simple Glaucoma (Left Eye)

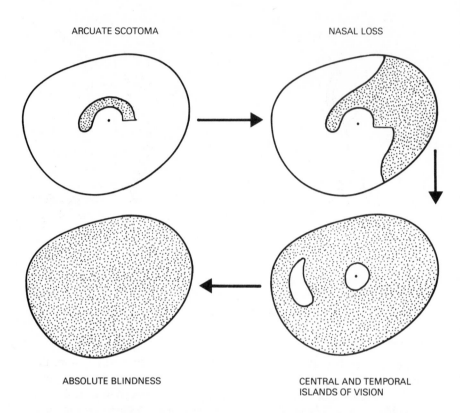

ARCUATE SCOTOMA

NASAL LOSS

ABSOLUTE BLINDNESS

CENTRAL AND TEMPORAL
ISLANDS OF VISION

incision in the sclera just behind the limbus and cauterising the wound edges. Aqueous drains through the incision into the subconjunctival space; here it raises a filtering bleb (which looks like a fluid-filled blister) from which the aqueous gradually disperses.

Trabeculectomy is currently a popular operation (Figure 16.4). Under local or general anaesthesia a lid retractor is inserted and the eye immobilised by a superior rectus stitch. An incision is made through both the conjunctiva and Tenon's capsule, well away from the limbus. These tissues are dissected off the sclera until the conjunctival flap can be reflected over the cornea. A square, partial thickness scleral flap is fashioned with a knife and then a block of tissue consisting of the deeper parts of the sclera and part of the trabecular meshwork is excised. The underlying iris is abscised as a peripheral iridectomy. The scleral flap is sutured back and the conjunctiva and Tenon's capsule meticulously repaired. The bleb created by this operation is more posterior, diffuse and less vulnerable to trauma than the bleb created by Scheie's operation.

Frequently, a drainage operation will permanently lower the intraocular press-

Figure 16.3: Scheie's Operation

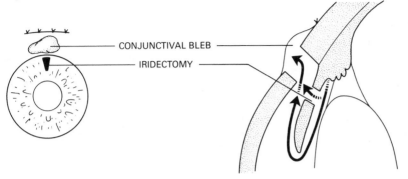

ure to normal levels, so reducing the need for patients to attend hospital so often. Sometimes supplementary medical treatment is necessary. Occasionally the operation fails.

Laser Trabeculoplasty

During the past few years it has been discovered that the intraocular pressure of many patients can be reduced by applying laser burns to the trabecular meshwork. This treatment is usually recommended for those patients who have

Figure 16.4: Trabeculectomy

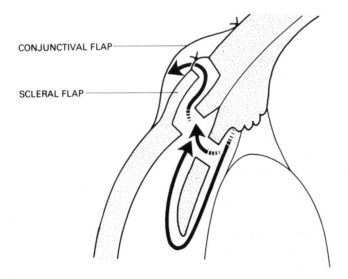

failed to respond to medical treatment, before conventional surgery is recommended. Laser trabeculoplasty is carried out as an out-patient procedure. The Argon Laser is mounted on a standard slit-lamp. After the instillation of local anaesthetic drops the surgeon places a gonioscope on the patient's eye and fires the laser between 50 to 100 times to create tiny burns around half the circumference of the trabecular meshwork. Initially, there may be a transitory rise in the intraocular pressure so the patient is usually asked to stay in the Department for about a couple of hours, so that the pressure may be checked again and treatment prescribed if necessary. It is not yet known precisely how this treatment works. Perhaps the burns cause local contraction of tissue which leads to adjacent parts of the trabecular meshwork opening up.

Post-operative Complications

1. The drainage of aqueous may be excessive in the early days, leading to a large bleb and 'flat' anterior chamber with the formation of choroidal detachments (Figure 16.5).

Figure 16.5: Choroidal Detachments

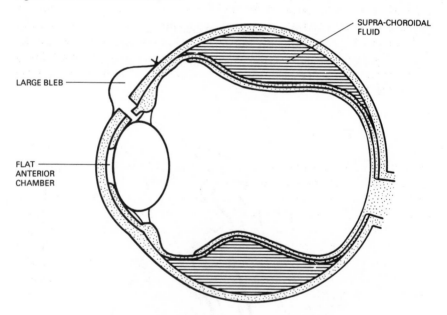

These are seen as dark balloons in the fundus, very similar in appearance to an extensive retinal detachment.

Management is by dilatation of the pupil, the prescription of acetazolamide to reduce aqueous production, and by firm padding and bandaging of the eye. Usually the anterior chamber deepens and the choroidal detachment resolves after a few days, presumably because scarring reduces the size of the surgical drainage channel. If the condition persists and the eye becomes inflamed, an operation is necessary in which the supra-choroidal fluid is drained and the anterior chamber is reformed. Occasionally the wound needs to be resutured.

2. Hyphaema.

3. Infection — panophthalmitis.

4. Rupture of the bleb is a late complication as the bleb walls become progressively thinned. The patient complains of blurred vision and a watery eye. The anterior chamber flattens and the intraocular pressure falls. Admission to hospital and treatment with antibiotic drops and firm bandaging of the eye may allow the eye to heal; but if the eye becomes infected it may be lost due to panophthalmitis.

Low-tension Glaucoma

In this condition there is cupping of the optic disc and progressive field loss in the presence of an intraocular pressure which lies within the normal range. It usually occurs in the elderly and may be due to vascular insufficiency of the optic nerve and retina which renders the eye vulnerable to even a normal intraocular pressure, or to such minor elevations as occur during the 24 hours. Treatment may be given to reduce the pressure to even lower levels, but it is often unsuccessful in halting the field loss.

Ocular Hypertension

Many individuals have a high intraocular pressure without disc cupping or field loss. If observed over many years, some (but not all) go on to develop chronic open angle glaucoma. Ophthalmologists vary in the way they manage such patients: all would wish to see these patients regularly to detect early cupping or field loss. Most would treat high pressures (30mm Hg or more) even without such changes. However, many surgeons feel that it is unreasonable to make patients suffer the side-effects of drops or tablets in order to reduce a slightly elevated pressure which has done no damage to the eye and which they feel may well not cause damage in the future.

Narrow-angle Glaucoma (Acute Angle-closure Glaucoma)

Mechanism

In this condition the peripheral part of the iris comes to lie up against the back of the adjacent part of the cornea. The angle thus becomes occluded and the intraocular pressure rises. The angle can be seen to be closed on gonioscopy (Figures 16.6 and 16.7).

Figure 16.6: Normal and Narrow Drainage Angle

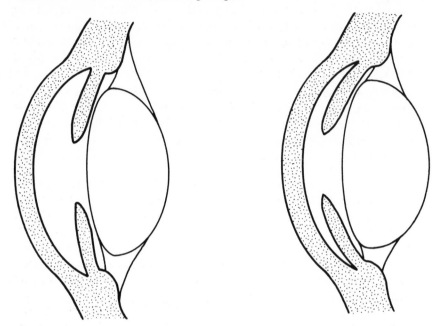

Figure 16.7: Gonioscopic Appearance of Normal and Narrow Angles

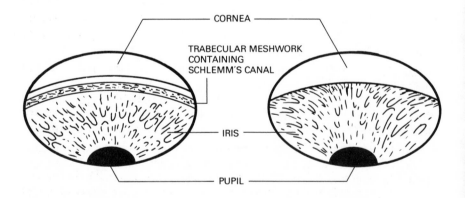

There appear to be two mechanisms of such angle occlusion. Both tend to occur in those patients who are hypermetropic. The eye is short; the anterior chamber is shallow; and the angle is consequently narrow.

Elderly patients are particularly at risk, for the lens increases in size during life and it moves progressively further forward with increasing age. Both these factors tend to lead to narrowing of the angle.

The more common reason for angle closure is the accumulation of aqueous behind the iris because there is an inadequate flow of aqueous through the pupil. This is especially likely to happen when the pupil is mid-dilated, when there is some obstruction to the flow of aqueous but whilst the iris is relatively flaccid and can be pushed forward. The patient typically experiences an attack whilst walking home from the pub or watching television in semi-darkness.

The less common cause of such angle closure is when the pupil of a patient at risk is dilated with a mydriatic. The iris bunches up peripherally and covers up the trabecular meshwork.

Signs and Symptoms

Usually one eye is affected first, but the second eye becomes involved sooner or later in most cases. At first the patient may experience reversible rises of intraocular pressure which may be precipitated by darkness. He develops a headache, an ache in the eye and blurred vision. The latter is due to corneal oedema as aqueous is forced into the cornea under pressure. Corneal oedema also causes the patient to see 'haloes' — rainbow coloured rings around bright lights. These attacks tend to resolve during sleep because the pupils then constrict.

Eventually an attack occurs which does not resolve spontaneously. Patients often do not present until this stage. There is extreme pain, blurred vision and sometimes vomiting. The eye is red, the cornea hazy, the pupil semi-dilated and unresponsive to light and the intraocular pressure is so high (60 to 70mm Hg) that the eye feels hard. If treatment is not quickly instituted, then permanent damage to the eye results. An anterior uveitis develops, peripheral anterior synechiae form, so that the angle is permanently closed (Figure 16.8). The optic disc becomes pale and cupped with partial or total loss of vision.

Diagnosis

This is fairly easy during an acute attack because of the characteristic symptoms and signs. At the stage of reversible episodes the diagnosis depends on the history, the finding of narrow angles on gonioscopy and the results of provocative tests as follows.

Prone Dark Room Test. The eye is examined on the slit-lamp and the intraocular pressure is recorded. The patient then lies prone in a darkened room with his eyes closed for 45 minutes. He must not go to sleep (this leads to the pupils constricting) so a relative may be asked to talk to him. The examination and pressure measurement are then repeated. A substantial increase in the pressure confirms the diagnosis of narrow-angle glaucoma.

Mydriatic Test. The intraocular pressures are recorded before and after the pupil is dilated with a weak mydriatic. A marked increase in pressure confirms

Figure 16.8: Peripheral Anterior Synechiae

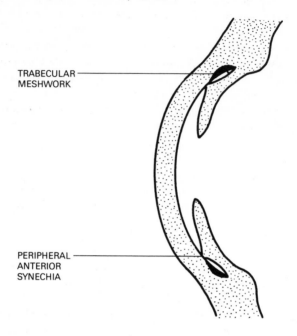

TRABECULAR
MESHWORK

PERIPHERAL
ANTERIOR
SYNECHIA

the diagnosis of narrow-angle glaucoma. Unfortunately, it may be difficult to reverse the provoked rise in pressure which has led to this test largely falling into disrepute.

Treatment

A patient suffering from reversible narrow angle attacks, confirmed by a prone dark room test, should be advised to have a peripheral iridectomy (or laser iridotomy) as soon as possible. This usually achieves a permanent cure as aqueous can pass directly into the anterior chamber via the iridectomy and so the tendency for the peripheral part of the iris to balloon forward (iris bombé) is eliminated (Figure 16.9). Pilocarpine drops are usually prescribed until the operation can be performed as they keep the pupils slightly constricted but they should never be advised as an alternative to surgery unless the patient is totally unfit for the operation because an acute attack may still occur in spite of their use.

The patient with an established attack should be admitted to hospital immediately. Acetazolamide (Diamox) 500mg is given intravenously and then 250mg orally four times daily to reduce aqueous formation and lower the intraocular pressure. Pilocarpine 4% is instilled intensively (e.g., at 10 to 15 minutes intervals) to constrict the pupil in an attempt to pull the iris out of the angle. Steroid drops are instilled to reduce the inflammation. Analgesics, antiemetics and the correction of dehydration are necessary in severe cases. The fellow eye is treated with pilocarpine 2% drops in the hope of protecting it from a similar attack.

After a few hours the patient is re-examined and the intraocular pressure measured. Early cases usually respond favourably to treatment by the return of the intraocular pressure to normal, the clearing of corneal oedema and the restoration of a small round pupil. The acetazolamide may then be stopped and treatment continued with pilocarpine and steroid drops until the eye is quiet. A peripheral iridectomy is then performed.

Figure 16.9: Peripheral Iridectomy

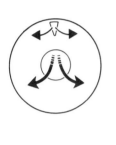
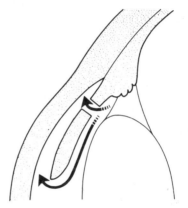

If there has been no improvement after a few hours (this is common when the condition has been present for days before the diagnosis was made), oral glycerol 50% (1.5 grams per kilogram of body weight) in fruit juice, or intravenous mannitol (200 mls of 20% solution) may be given to dehydrate the eye. In some cases the pupil remains semi-dilated and the intraocular pressure rises as soon as the acetazolamide and the osmotic diuretics are stopped. This is because the drainage angle has been permanently closed by peripheral anterior synechiae. Some surgeons opt for a drainage operation (e.g., trabeculectomy) to provide an alternative route by which aqueous may escape from the eye. Others favour the more conservative approach of an initial iridectomy and subsequent medical treatment.

Follow-up Treatment

The fellow eye is nearly always at risk of an attack of acute glaucoma and it is vital to prevent this as the first eye may have suffered considerable damage. It is usual to perform a peripheral iridectomy on the second eye before the patient leaves hospital. Steroid drops are given for a couple of weeks after discharge and the patient is followed up in the clinic. If the intraocular pressures remain normal and the patient is symptom free, then six-monthly visits are adequate. Some cases, with permanent angle damage, continue to require medical treatment to control the pressure

Malignant Glaucoma (Ciliary Block Glaucoma)

This is a rare complication of glaucoma operations. The anterior chamber is 'flat' and the intraocular pressure is very high (Figure 16.10). It is particularly likely to follow drainage surgery on an eye chronically affected by angle closure.

Intensive dilatation of the pupil may correct some cases. Otherwise, the drainage of aqueous that has become trapped within the vitreous, together with the reformation of the anterior chamber with air, should reverse the abnormality.

Figure 16.10: Malignant Glaucoma

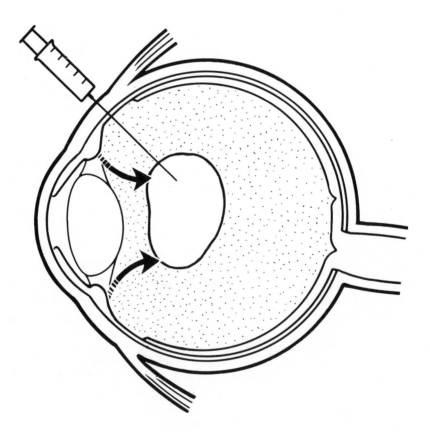

Congenital Glaucoma (Buphthalmos)

This is a rare and serious condition affecting one or both eyes of babies. It may be part of a syndrome with other ocular abnormalities (e.g., Sturge-Weber syndrome). Characteristically a layer of abnormal tissue overlies the trabecular meshwork.

The infant's eye is elastic and so a raised intraocular pressure causes the globe to enlarge. Later, the optic disc becomes pale and cupped. The cornea is hazy due to oedema and splits occur in Descemet's membrane. Refractive errors develop because of the altered shape of the eye and the abnormal position of the lens.

Signs and Symptoms

Parents or doctors may notice the large size of the child's eye. Commonly, however, the diagnosis becomes apparent only when the cornea becomes hazy and the child is manifestly photophobic.

Management

Immediate admission to hospital and examination under anaesthesia should be advised. The corneal diameter is measured and a refraction and inspection of the fundi and gonioscopy are performed if the cornea is sufficiently clear to allow these procedures to be carried out. (Removal of the corneal epithelium may improve the view of the fundus.) Finally, the intraocular pressure is measured with a hand-held applanation (Perkins) tonometer.

Treatment

The prime treatment in most cases is the incision of the abnormal tissue in the angle by goniotomy (dividing the angle). Goniotomy should be performed under general anaesthesia (Figure 16.11). A Koeppe contact lens enables the surgeon to see the drainage angle through the operating microscope. A goniotomy knife is inserted at the limbus, passed across the anterior chamber and used to incise a quadrant of the abnormal drainage angle. Complications of goniotomy include damage to the lens and hyphaema.

A further examination under anaesthesia (EUA) is made once the eye has healed. If the intraocular pressure is still high a further goniotomy may be performed in another quadrant. Once the condition is stable, three-monthly EUAs are arranged. Refraction, the prescription of glasses and the treatment of associated amblyopia by patching are as vital as the control of the intraocular pressure if the child's vision is to be preserved.

Figure 16.11: Goniotomy

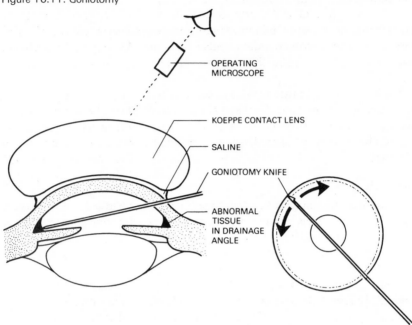

OPERATING
MICROSCOPE

KOEPPE CONTACT LENS

SALINE

GONIOTOMY KNIFE

ABNORMAL
TISSUE
IN DRAINAGE
ANGLE

Secondary Glaucoma

Glaucoma may complicate an anterior uveitis when the inflammation has led to the margin of the pupil becoming adherent to the anterior lens capsule. Such ring synechiae prevent aqueous passing forwards through the pupil and iris bombé results (chapter 15). This further contributes to the glaucoma by causing angle closure. Alternatively, the uveitis may lead to exudate blocking the angle. In chronic cases, the angle becomes occluded by the formation of peripheral anterior synechiae.

Thrombotic Glaucoma (Rubeotic Glaucoma)

This most commonly occurs about three months after a central retinal vein occlusion (100 day glaucoma) or occasionally in patients with proliferative diabetic retinopathy. The angle is blocked by new vessels which arise because of hypoxia within the eye.

A central retinal vein occlusion may be the presenting feature of, or occur in a patient with, chronic open-angle glaucoma. Hence, a patient with neovascular glaucoma in one eye should have the fellow eye carefully checked for any evidence of chronic open-angle disease.

Signs and Symptoms

The eye is red, painful, and nearly blind (a visual acuity of counting fingers or less is typical). Corneal oedema may obscure the abnormal vessels on the iris and in the angle. The intraocular pressure is characteristically very high (greater than 70mm Hg).

Management

There is no cure. The aim is to relieve pain. Mydriatic and steroid drops may provide such relief. A retrobulbar injection of 70% alcohol, which may be performed as an Out-patient procedure, is more likely to relieve severe pain but the injection accelerates the inevitable loss of vision. If this approach fails, then enucleation may be the only answer. It is best delayed until the patient requests it.

If thrombotic glaucoma occurs in the only seeing eye a drainage operation may be justified; it is more risky and is less likely to control the pressure than in chronic open angle glaucoma; but if it succeeds then the otherwise inevitable absolute blindness may be prevented.

Steroid-induced Glaucoma

Some patients develop high intraocular pressures after a few weeks of treatment with steroid drops (or rarely, systemic steroids). The pressure falls when treatment is discontinued but glaucomatous damage may have occurred. Local steroids should never be prescribed without close ophthalmic supervision.

Dislocated Lens and Glaucoma (see chapter 17)

Aphakic Glaucoma

Glaucoma may be diagnosed for the first time after cataract extraction. Causes include post-operative uveitis, steroid-induced glaucoma or previously undiagnosed chronic open-angle glaucoma.

17 THE LENS

Age Changes

The lens continues to grow throughout life. New fibres are deposited beneath the capsule; older fibres are pushed inwards to form a compact nucleus. With increasing age the nucleus becomes larger and harder; this tends to make the eye more myopic. The enlargement of the lens causes a gradual shallowing of the anterior chamber. Opacities in either the cortex or the nucleus commonly develop in later life. Cataract is another name for lens opacity.

Cataract

Causes

Senile cataracts are the most common and are the easiest to treat. Congenital cataracts may be hereditary or be due to intrauterine infections (e.g., rubella). Trauma, whether blunt, penetrating or due to an intraocular foreign body, commonly causes lens opacities. Young diabetics occasionally develop cataracts; older diabetics frequently have senile cataracts. Lens opacities commonly develop in eyes affected by chronic uveitis or in patients with retinitis pigmentosa. Finally, drugs (e.g., steroids), heat and irradiation may also cause lens opacities.

Signs and Symptoms

The main complaint is of gradual loss of vision. Sometimes cataracts also cause diplopia and lead to patients seeing haloes. With a nuclear opacity the patient may see better in the dark because the pupil then dilates slightly so allowing light to pass through the clear cortex (Figure 17.1). Such patients may be helped by the use of mydriatic drops so that the pupils are kept permanently dilated. Early lens opacities may be seen with the ophthalmoscope as dark shadows against the red reflex, or with the slit-lamp as white opacities.

Later, the whole lens becomes milky white, obliterating the red reflex and totally obscuring the fundus view; this is a mature cataract. Very rarely a mature cataract will swell up and cause angle-closure glaucoma or leak lens protein, so causing a uveitis. Only then will the patient experience any pain.

Management

Some surgeons consider it advisable to remove a mature cataract to prevent lens-induced glaucoma or uveitis but the main reason for removing a cataract is to restore vision. Only rarely does a patient seek removal of a cataract to rid himself

146

Figure 17.1: Lens Opacities: a. Nuclear; b. Cortical

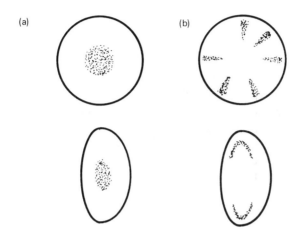

of the unsightliness of a white pupil. A cataract can only be dispersed by removal of the lens. There is no known way of dissolving lens opacities by medical means.

Without the lens the eye is very long-sighted and the patient is unable to accommodate for near vision. No method of optical correction restores completely normal vision and each method of correction has disadvantages (see below). It is usually best to defer operation until the patient's vision has fallen sufficiently to impair his life-style considerably. Many patients can read adequately and can manage everyday tasks with an acuity of 6/24 in either eye. However, those who wish to drive need a binocular acuity of at least 6/15 and an adequate field of vision. Regular Out-patient visits are important so that the Ophthalmologist can ensure that visual deterioration is due solely to the cataracts and not to the development of other conditions (e.g., glaucoma) which might require treatment. Patients may be helped by the prescription of new spectacles, as lens opacities are often accompanied by refractive changes; and the effect of mydriatic drops can be assessed.

Children with cataracts pose special problems. Amblyopia, squint (chapter 18) and nystagmus may develop if cataracts become dense. Cataract surgery in the young is usually more hazardous than in the elderly. Sometimes an optical iridectomy (Figure 17.2) provides adequate visual improvement without the risk of cataract surgery.

Patients with other eye problems, e.g., diabetes, glaucoma or uveitis, are less likely to have a good visual result from surgery and, consequently, an operation should be less readily undertaken. Finally, patients must be medically fit for operation whether under local or general anaesthesia. If a local anaesthetic is chosen, the patient should be calm, co-operative and, preferably, have reasonable hearing.

Figure 17.2: Optical Iridectomy

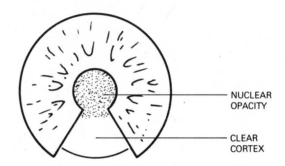

NUCLEAR
OPACITY

CLEAR
CORTEX

Pre-operative Care

Most patients are admitted the day before operation. The eyes are re-examined to exclude any infection or other problem contra-indicating surgery. A general examination is performed by the House Surgeon and the patient is seen by the anaesthetist. A consent form must be signed and the eye to be operated upon identified by a mark on the forehead. The pupil is dilated, antibiotic drops instilled four-hourly and the eye lashes may be cut short. A mannitol infusion or Diamox injection is sometimes given shortly before the induction of anaesthesia in order to reduce the intraocular pressure.

If a local anaesthetic is required, cocaine drops are instilled whilst the patient is still on the ward. A facial block, retrobulbar injection, infiltration of the lids and around the insertion of the superior rectus muscle are performed in theatre after skin preparation and draping (chapter 8).

Intracapsular Cataract Extraction

The lids and peri-orbital skin are cleaned with an aqueous solution of antiseptic. Sterile towels are used to wrap the head firmly and cover the face and the other eye. Antibiotic drops are instilled. Adrenaline drops are used to minimise bleeding provided the anaesthetist permits their use. The lids are retracted with lid sutures clipped to the head towels or with a light speculum. A superior rectus suture is used to fixate the eye (Figure 17.3). If the palpebral aperture is very small an incision at the other canthus will enlarge it. This is called a lateral canthotomy.

The eye may be opened with a von Graefe knife (Figure 17.4). The eye is punctured temporally, the blade passed across the anterior chamber to emerge nasally, and then a semi-circular cut made to complete the incision. A small conjunctival flap is fashioned during the completion of the manoeuvre.

Nowadays an 'ab externo' incision is more often used (Figure 17.5). The conjunctival flap is fashioned first, then a groove made outside the limbus with a

Figure 17.3: Lid Sutures and Superior Rectus Stitch

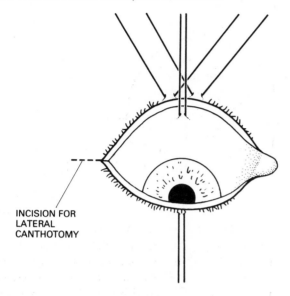

INCISION FOR
LATERAL
CANTHOTOMY

Figure 17.4: von Graefe Section

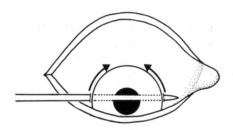

Figure 17.5: Ab Externo Incision

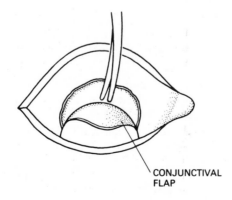

CONJUNCTIVAL
FLAP

blade and the incision completed either with the blade or with scissors. Aqueous humour escapes when the eye is opened. Several sutures of either virgin silk or monofilament nylon are then inserted, but not tied, and looped out of the way. A peripheral iridectomy is performed. Up to 0.5 ml of 1 in 5000 solution of alpha-chymotrypsin is injected into the posterior chamber through the iridectomy in order to dissolve the zonule which is holding the lens in place. After three minutes it is washed out with saline (Figure 17.6).

Figure 17.6: The Eye Ready for Lens Extraction

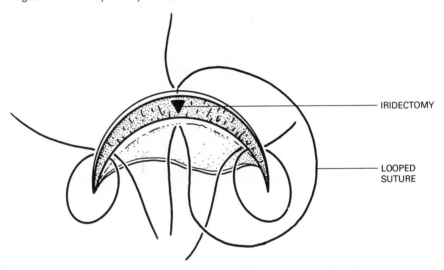

IRIDECTOMY

LOOPED
SUTURE

The lens may be extracted with a cryoprobe, forceps or an erisophake. The assistant grasps the conjunctival flap, thus retracting the cornea; the iris is retracted with a brush, sponge or forceps and the cryoprobe, for example, applied to the upper pole of the lens. In addition, pressure may be applied inferiorly with a squint hook. (Figure 17.7).

As soon as the lens is delivered the eye is closed; the iris is replaced, if necessary, with a brush or iris repositor; the pupil is constricted with pilocarpine drops or acetylcholine injection (Miochol) and the sutures tied. Additional sutures are inserted until the eye is water-tight. If necessary, the anterior chamber is reformed with saline. Antibiotic drops are instilled; the conjunctival flap may be sutured with collagen. The eye is closed and padded. The upper lid sutures may be taped down to the cheek to close the eye; this is particularly important if a facial nerve block has been used for the sphincter-like action of the orbicularis oculi is impaired. A pad and cartella shield are taped over the lids.

Figure 17.7: Lens Extraction

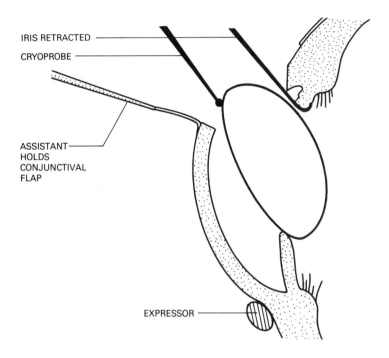

IRIS RETRACTED

CRYOPROBE

ASSISTANT
HOLDS
CONJUNCTIVAL
FLAP

EXPRESSOR

Extracapsular Cataract Extraction

In young people the posterior lens capsule is firmly attached to the vitreous face. If an intracapsular cataract extraction is attempted vitreous is likely to be lost, so an extracapsular technique (in which most of the capsule is left behind) should be chosen. The eye is opened, and the anterior capsule is torn and removed with forceps; the lens nucleus is expressed and removed with a vectis (Figure 17.8). The cortical lens matter is removed by irrigation with saline. Of course, alpha-chymotrypsin is not used in this operation (Figure 17.9).

In theory all cataracts can be removed by the extracapsular technique. As with any operation on the eye, good results are obtained only if meticulous care is taken. If soft lens matter is left behind, it swells post-operatively and becomes opaque. It may block the pupil and also cause iritis. Mydriatic and steroid drops should be used frequently until the lens matter is absorbed. The posterior lens capsule may become thickened and opaque and impair vision. Then a second operation to make a hole in the posterior capsule (capsulotomy) may be necessary.

Figure 17.8: Vectis

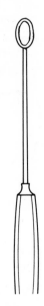

Figure 17.9: The Eye at the End of Extracapsular Cataract Extraction

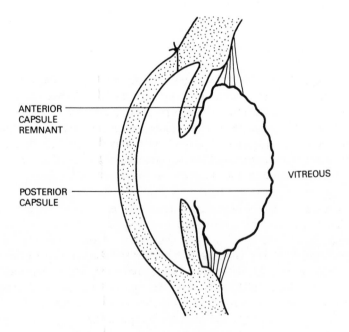

ANTERIOR
CAPSULE
REMNANT

POSTERIOR
CAPSULE

VITREOUS

Posterior Capsulotomy

The pupil is widely dilated and the eye immobilised. A Ziegler knife is used to puncture the eye at the limbus and then incise the capsule in the pupillary area. Only a small gap is required for good vision (Figure 17.10). Alternatively, a capsulotomy may be carried out with a laser.

Figure 17.10: Posterior Capsulotomy

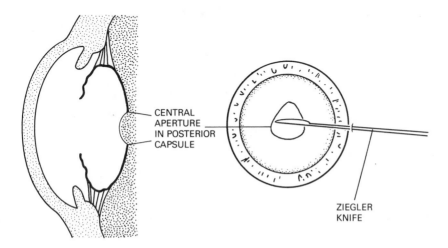

Lens Aspiration

The lens of a child does not have a hard nucleus and the whole contents of the lens are soluble. A congenital cataract may be treated, first by discission (tearing open the anterior lens capsule with a sharp needle) and then washing out the lens protein with Ringer solution. These manoeuvres may be performed through a puncture at the limbus and the anterior chamber kept deep by a continuous infusion of Ringer saline through another puncture site (Figure 17.11). The posterior capsule is not touched. A capsulotomy may be required later.

Lensectomy

There are now available instruments which combine the facility to irrigate the inside of the eye, through infusion and aspiration tubes, and have as well a cutting tip. Such an instrument is ideal for removing cataracts in childhood, a procedure that is known as lensectomy. In those children with juvenile arthritis (Still's disease) who develop a chronic uveitis and cataracts, this approach is to be preferred, for it is the best way to remove all the soft lens matter. Some

Figure 17.11: Lens Aspiration

(a)

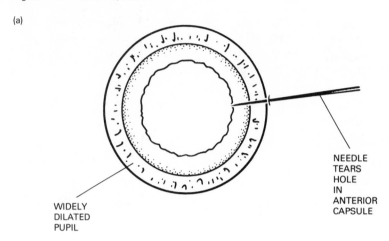

NEEDLE
TEARS
HOLE
IN
ANTERIOR
CAPSULE

WIDELY
DILATED
PUPIL

(b)

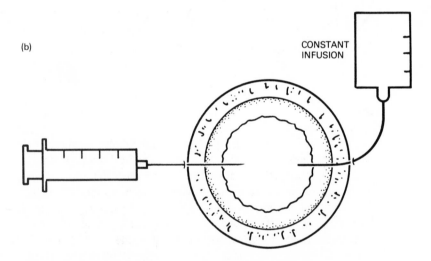

CONSTANT
INFUSION

surgeons prefer to remove the posterior capsule and some vitreous as well.

Phako Emulsification

The adult lens nucleus can often be aspirated if it has first been emulsified by an ultrasonic probe introduced through a small limbal incision (an anterior capsulotomy must be performed first). This is phako-emulsification — another extracapsular technique. Unfortunately, the equipment is very expensive and some lens nuclei are too hard to emulsify, so phako-emulsification is not widely performed.

Corneal Section (Figure 17.12)

Lens extraction may be performed through a corneal incision rather than through a limbal incision.

Figure 17.12: Corneal and Limbal Incisions

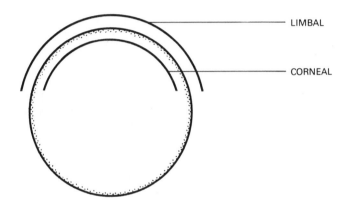

LIMBAL

CORNEAL

Operative Complications

Bleeding

Bleeding from the iris into the anterior chamber is common. It usually stops spontaneously and the blood can often be removed by irrigation.

Vitreous Loss

This may occur at the time of extracting the lens during an intracapsular extraction or if the posterior capsule is inadvertently ruptured during an extracapsular extraction. Loss of solid vitreous is more serious than loss of fluid vitreous. It occurs more commonly in young patients and in those who are myopic. There is a risk of retinal detachment or macular oedema developing following vitreous loss. It is therefore important to avoid vitreous loss by preventing undue pressure on the eye from a speculum or any other instrument and by reducing the bulk of the vitreous with mannitol given pre-operatively to those at particular risk of vitreous being lost.

If vitreous loss occurs it is important that the wound be completely cleared before the eye is closed. An anterior vitrectomy must be carried out with a vitrectomy instrument or by mopping up the fluid vitreous with dry sponges and cutting any strands with scissors. The wound is painted with hyaluronidase (Hyalase). This enzyme dissolves the formed vitreous and aids cleaning of the wound edges. In addition, fluid vitreous may be aspirated from the centre of the eye with a wide bore needle; this allows solid vitreous to fall back into the eye (Figure 17.13). Unless cleared, vitreous remnants may gradually draw the iris up into the wound (hammock pupil — Figure 17.14).

Figure 17.13: Anterior Vitrectomy

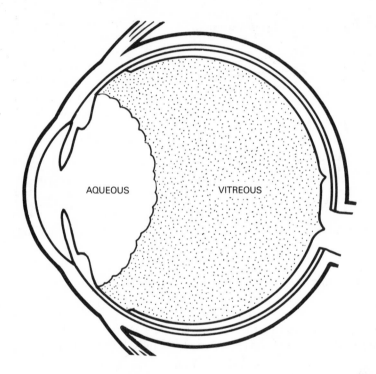

Capsule Rupture

This may occur during either intracapsular or extracapsular surgery. In the former instance, the bulk of the lens can usually be removed with the cryoprobe but fragments of capsule and soft lens matter may need to be removed by irrigation or with forceps. Post-operatively the eye should be treated as for a planned extracapsular operation.

Lens Dislocation (Figure 17.15)

Occasionally the lens dislocates inferiorly during its attempted removal. It can usually be retrieved with a vectis.

Figure 17.14: Hammock Pupil

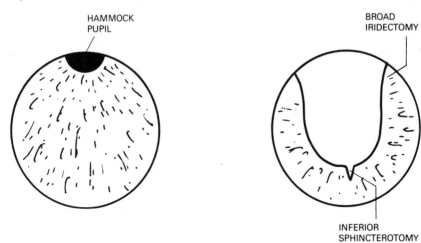

HAMMOCK
PUPIL

BROAD
IRIDECTOMY

INFERIOR
SPHINCTEROTOMY

Figure 17.15: Lens Dislocation

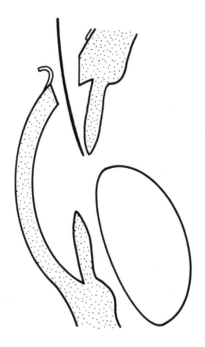

Expulsive Haemorrhage (Figure 17.16)

A choroidal haemorrhage occurs rarely during cataract surgery. The lens, vit-

Figure 17.16: Expulsive Haemorrhage

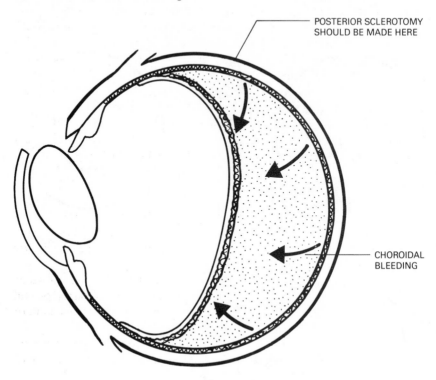

POSTERIOR SCLEROTOMY
SHOULD BE MADE HERE

CHOROIDAL
BLEEDING

reous and retina may be completely expelled from the eye. The surgeon may attempt to release the blood, which is expelling the contents of the eye, by making puncture wounds in the posterior parts of the sclera.

Post-operative Management

Patients are usually nursed flat on their backs (unlike most post-operative patients). They are kept quiet, and in most hospitals remain in bed for the first day. Analgesics, such as Pethidine, are rarely required. Severe post-operative pain should be reported to the doctor in charge straight away; it may be due to infection or raised intraocular pressure. A normal diet may be given but the patient should avoid tough food like apples, toffee or steak. Bed baths are only necessary for the first couple of days. Patients should initially be shaved by a nurse. Normal visiting is allowed except on the day of operation.

The *First Dressing* is carried out on the morning after the operation. Ideally both the doctor and the nurse should examine the patient together. The procedure is explained to the patient and he is asked to keep his hands away from his face. After washing her hands, the nurse removes the cartella shield and the pad and cleans the patient's eye with gauze dipped in saline. Any lid sutures are cut and removed. The patient should be asked to open both eyes. If necessary, the lids can be gently retracted by drawing the skin of the lids over the orbital margins. With the aid of a light from a torch (and magnifying glasses if necessary) the following details are noted:

1. *Discharge.* Purulent matter on the lids or pad is a sign of infection.
2. *Lids.* Excessive swelling or redness of the lids may be due to infection or allergy.
3. *Conjunctiva.* Chemosis may be due to infection or to a leaking wound.
4. *Wound.* Abnormal signs include gaping of the wound edges, iris prolapse and pus in the wound.
5. *Cornea.* This should be clear and bright like a mirror. Any dullness may be a warning of infection or raised intraocular pressure. Some cloudiness near the wound is a common result of manipulation of the cornea during surgery, particularly after a corneal section. Clearer lines may be seen within the cloudy area; this is termed striate keratitis.
6. *Anterior chamber.* This should be of a normal depth. Shallowing or absence of the anterior chamber denotes a leaking wound or pupil block. A partial or total hyphaema may be present. An hypopyon is a warning sign of infection or severe uveitis.
7. *Pupil.* This should be round and central. Minor degrees of irregularity result from trauma to the iris during surgery. An updrawn pupil may be the pointer to an iris prolapse (Figure 17.17).
8. *Red reflex.* The ocular media should be clear enough to permit a red reflex to be seen with an ophthalmoscope.

Figure 17.17: Iris Prolapse

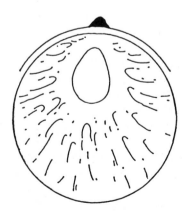

If the first dressing is satisfactory, the pad may be left off by day and the patient is given glasses to wear. Temporary glasses containing a +10 dioptre sphere (sometimes as Fresnel lenses, see Figure 17.20) give a welcome improvement in vision to many patients. Otherwise dark glasses may be used to relieve the photophobia associated with dilatation of the pupil. The eye is padded at night. Mydriatic and steroid-antibiotic drops are instilled several times daily. These prevent the formation of posterior synechiae and control post-operative uveitis.

Patients are discharged after a few days, ideally to a convalescent home or to caring relatives. They are supplied with temporary or dark glasses to be used by day and a cartella shield to wear at night. The same drops are continued at home. Some weeks absence from work is recommended and heavy work in the house or garden is not allowed during that time. Travelling on buses is best avoided at first, for the patient may bang his eye if he stumbles as he tries to reach a seat on a moving bus. The patient's hair should only be back washed for the six weeks after operation.

Patients are seen in the clinic two weeks after discharge to check that the eye is healing satisfactorily. At a second appointment four weeks later, a refraction is carried out and glasses or contact lenses are prescribed if necessary (see below). If all is well the drops are stopped and restrictions lifted but the patient is followed up in the clinic first three months and then six months later in case the spectacles need changing or late complications develop.

Post-operative Complications

Infection — Panophthalmitis

This is a disaster as infection spreads rapidly throughout the eye. Occasionally the infection is localised to the vitreous cavity (endophthalmitis). Typically, patients complain of severe pain at the first dressing. There is a purulent discharge; swelling of the lids, chemosis, haziness of the cornea and an hypopyon may be present.

Immediate action must be taken to identify the infecting organism and to treat the eye with antibiotic and anti-inflammatory agents. The drug regime given in Table 17.1 is instituted. As soon as possible the patient is taken to theatre and under general anaesthesia, specimens of aqueous and vitreous humour are aspirated and used to prepare Gram-stained smears, agar plates and broth cultures. Pars plana vitrectomy (chapter 18) followed by intravitreal antibiotic injections gives the best chance of controlling the infection. If a vitrectomy instrument is not available, intravitreal antibiotic injection alone may suffice. A subconjunctival antibiotic injection can be given at the end of the procedure.

Despite early diagnosis and treatment, the eye may be largely destroyed by the inflammation so that no useful sight remains. Some eyes have to be eviscerated to prevent spread of infection to the central nervous system and blood stream.

Table 17.1: Treatment of Panophthalmitis

a) Topical	concentrated gentamicin drops (15mg/ml) hourly.
b) Intravenous	gentamicin 100-200 mgs 8 hourly. cloxacillin 1-2 grams 6 hourly.
c) Subconjunctival	gentamicin 40 mgs. methicillin 150 mgs — repeated within 12 hours.
d) Intravitreal	gentamicin 0.2 mgs — 0.4 mgs. methicillin 2 mgs.

Note: Gentamicin and methicillin must not be mixed in the same syringe.

Iris Prolapse (Figure 17.17)

This is treated by immediate re-operation to abscise or replace the prolapsed iris and resuture the wound.

Pupil Block (Figure 17.18)

After intracapsular cataract extraction, the pupil margin may adhere to the vitreous, particularly if there is marked post-operative inflammation. If the entire periphery of the pupil margin is bound down to the vitreous face, then aqueous can no longer pass from the posterior chamber behind to the anterior chamber in front. This causes 'pupil block'. The aqueous consequently becomes pent up behind the iris. The iris is pushed forward and the anterior chamber becomes either shallow or 'flat'. The intraocular pressure rises and the patient complains of pain. Mydriatic and steroid drops are routinely given to prevent this complication. A peripheral iridectomy performed at the time of cataract extraction provides an extra exit for aqueous from the posterior chamber.

Sometimes these precautions fail, despite the presence of a peripheral iridectomy, because it too is occluded by the post-operative inflammation. Urgent treatment is then necessary. Intensive mydriatric drops, heat and a subconjunctival injection of mydricaine may be sufficient to break the pupillary adhesions and rectify the problem. Otherwise, re-operation to create a new peripheral iridectomy, or the creation of a laser iridotomy, is required.

High Intraocular Pressure

This may occur without the signs of pupil block. It is generally due to impaired outflow of aqueous through the trabecular meshwork in the immediate post-operative period. It subsides spontaneously. Acetazolamide is usually given for the first few days after surgery in these cases.

Leaking Wound

A poorly sutured wound may lead to an iris prolapse or to the continual leakage of aqueous from the eye. The anterior chamber is shallow or flat, the intraocular

Figure 17.18: Pupil Block

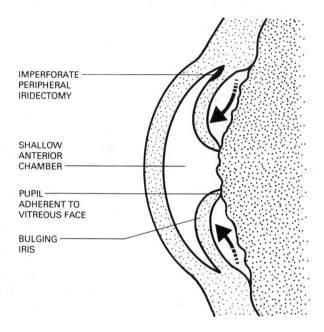

IMPERFORATE
PERIPHERAL
IRIDECTOMY

SHALLOW
ANTERIOR
CHAMBER

PUPIL
ADHERENT TO
VITREOUS FACE

BULGING
IRIS

pressure low and the conjunctiva is often oedematous. The leak is confirmed by instilling fluorescein into the conjunctival sac and looking for the area where it is diluted and becomes green due to the outflow of aqueous; this is Seidel's test. A few days of firm bandaging may allow healing to occur; otherwise resuturing is necessary.

Allergy

Drops, ointment or impregnated tulle may cause swelling of the lids, and redness and itching of the affected skin. Atropine and neomycin and certain preparations used as preservatives in drops are often to blame. The offending treatment should be withdrawn and another instituted. Hydrocortisone lotion will reduce the symptoms.

Remnants of Soft Lens Matter and Capsule

These may be present after planned extracapsular extraction or after the capsule has ruptured during intracapsular surgery. They are more apparent at first dressing than at the time of surgery. White opacities are noticed in the anterior chamber or pupil and the eye is often inflamed. Treatment is given as for planned extracapsular surgery (see p.151).

Retinal Detachment

This occasionally develops weeks, months or even years after cataract extraction (see chapter 19).

Optical Correction

The aphakic eye is very hypermetropic and has no power of accommodation for near vision (chapter 3; Figure 17.19). This hypermetropia is most simply corrected with a convex lens of about 10 dioptres power (Figure 17.20). Reading glasses (or bifocals) of about 13 dioptre power will also be necessary. Such spectacles may give good visual acuity yet they have many disadvantages. The lenses are thick and heavy and the spectacles tend to slip down the patient's nose. Lenticular or plastic lenses are not so heavy but lenticular lenses look unsightly and plastic lenses scratch easily. Fresnel lenses are very light and useful as temporary glasses but they do not give the best visual acuity. Because a spectacle lens is several millimetres in front of the pupil, a magnified and distorted image with reduced visual field and a ring scotoma is produced (Figure 17.21). For these reasons, patients are often better off with a moderately dense cataract reducing vision to 6/24, than with a spectacle corrected aphakic vision of 6/12 or so.

Figure 17.19: Aphakia

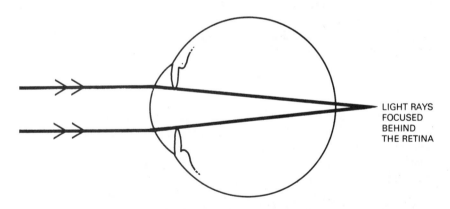

LIGHT RAYS
FOCUSED
BEHIND
THE RETINA

If only one eye is aphakic and the other has good vision, further problems exist. A +10 dioptre sphere lens in front of the aphakic eye will produce a retinal image 30 per cent larger than the retinal image in the fellow eye. It is impossible for the brain to fuse these two images and the patient will have diplopia. It is usually only worth operating on a patient with a unilateral cataract if the patient is to have an intraocular lens inserted or subsequently be fitted with a contact lens.

Figure 17.20: Spectacle Correction in Aphakia

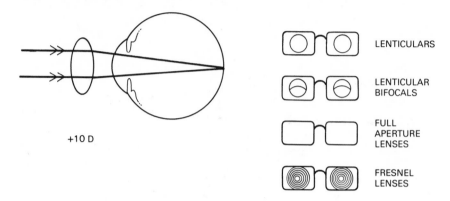

+10 D

LENTICULARS

LENTICULAR
BIFOCALS

FULL
APERTURE
LENSES

FRESNEL
LENSES

Figure 17.21: Visual Field in Spectacle Corrected Aphakia

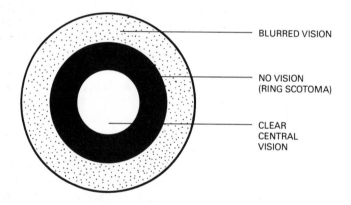

BLURRED VISION

NO VISION
(RING SCOTOMA)

CLEAR
CENTRAL
VISION

Because a contact lens is much nearer to the pupil than a spectacle lens, much less magnification of the retinal image results, so there should be no diplopia when the other eye is phakic (Figure 17.22). The visual field is not reduced by a contact lens and ordinary reading glasses can be used. Hard or soft, haptic or corneal lenses may be prescribed. However, contact lenses are difficult for the elderly to manipulate and many patients cannot tolerate them. Extended wear soft contact lenses are now available. They avoid the need for manipulation but need close medical supervision.

Intraocular lenses provide the best optical correction of aphakia, since they are sited within the eye and therefore introduce no element of magnification (Figure 17.23). The patient enjoys a full field of vision. Many surgeons aim to leave the patient slightly short-sighted so that he can read moderate size print without glasses. Clearly, in this instance the patient needs to wear a myopic correction for perfect distant vision and reading glasses to read fine print. There is,

Figure 17.22: Contact Lens Correction of Aphakia

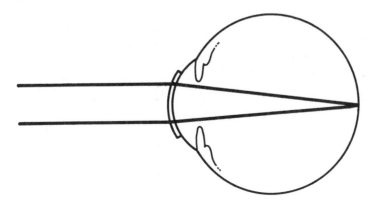

of course, none of the inconvenience associated with fitting, cleaning and wearing a contact lens. If spectacles do need to be worn, they are not of a high power and patients do not have trouble with them. This is in strict contrast to the plight of many patients with 'cataract' (aphakic) spectacles.

The ingenuity of eye surgeons is such that innumerable varieties of intraocular implants are already on the market and more are being designed. However, they are essentially of three types.

Anterior chamber implants. These are placed in the anterior chamber so that their supporting struts, or feet, lie on the scleral spur. They should remain stable within the eye for otherwise they will cause a low-grade uveitis, damage the trabecular meshwork and thus cause glaucoma, or precipitate recurrent bleeding in the eye. This complex of uveitis, glaucoma and hyphaema has led to the use of the term the 'UGH' syndrome. The corneal endothelium, too, may suffer and if its function is sufficiently impaired, then bullous keratopathy may develop. A rigid lens may lead to the eye being painful when rubbed. Consequently, lenses with flexible feet have been developed. These have the possible additional advantage of adapting to the dimensions of the eye so that they stabilise themselves but these flexible feet, or the material bonding them to the body of the lens (the optic), may undergo biodegradation and so cause problems in the long term. These lenses are usually inserted at the time of intracapsular cataract extraction but they may also be inserted as a secondary procedure in those patients who have undergone cataract surgery and who subsequently find that they cannot cope with either cataract glasses or contact lenses.

Iris supported lenses. An intracapsular extraction may be performed and a lens 'clipped' on to the iris by two or more loops lying on the anterior surface of the iris and others lying on its posterior surface. If the pupil dilates the implant tends to dislocate, so patients initially need to instil pilocarpine four times a day which many find irksome. In time, adhesions develop between the pupil margin and the

Figure 17.23: Intraocular Lenses for Aphakia

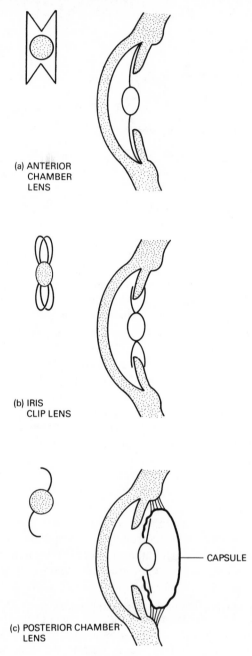

(a) ANTERIOR
     CHAMBER
     LENS

(b) IRIS
     CLIP LENS

(c) POSTERIOR CHAMBER
     LENS

CAPSULE

adjacent parts of the implant so that the pilocarpine can be stopped. The design of the implant is such that the pupil is square or otherwise distorted which many patients dislike. The bound-down pupil poses great problems should there later be a need to inspect the fundus fully, as when a retinal detachment or diabetic retinopathy develops. An iris clip lens tends to swing forwards and backwards on rotation of the eye and this may be associated with both corneal decompensation and macular oedema.

One way of trying to stabilise such a lens is to perform an extracapsular cataract extraction so that the posterior capsule remains intact. The implant is now described as receiving irido-capsular support.

Posterior chamber lenses. One great advantage of having the implant behind the iris is that it is well clear of both the corneal endothelium and the angle structures. It is necessary to carry out an extracapsular extraction so that the implant lies in the 'capsular bag'. If the bag ruptures, either at the time of surgery or later, the implant may fall into the vitreous cavity. The extracapsular technique, particularly in the the hands of the inexperienced, necessitates considerable irrigation of the anterior chamber and this itself can damage the corneal endothelium. The remaining posterior capsule may thicken and depress vision. However, the presence of an unthickened capsule is probably an advantage. The incidence of retinal detachment is probably less than is the case with the intracapsular technique. Hence there are particularly strong arguments for leaving the posterior capsule intact in patients who are myopic, have had a retinal tear or retinal detachment in either eye, or who have suffered trauma to the eye in the past. Because, until middle age, the vitreous is adherent to the lens, the young adult, too, should undergo extracapsular surgery. It is claimed that an intact posterior capsule also reduces the likelihood of macular oedema developing.

The surgeon should weigh up the pros and cons of each technique in any particular set of circumstances. He should then opt for what, in his hands, gives the best results.

Dislocated Lenses (Figure 17.24 and 17.25)

The suspensory ligament may be weakened by trauma, age, myopia or congenital defects (e.g., Marfan's syndrome). Incomplete rupture of the ligament causes the lens to subluxate (move and tilt); complete rupture causes the lens to dislocate either anteriorly (into the anterior chamber) or posteriorly (into the vitreous cavity).

A subluxated lens causes poor vision, refractive errors and sometimes monocular diplopia. Anterior dislocation is an emergency as the pupil becomes blocked by the lens and the intraocular pressure rises. Posterior dislocation causes poor vision due to loss of the lens from the pupillary area. Glaucoma sometimes develops but this may be due to the underlying cause of the dislocation (e.g., trauma).

Figure 17.24: Subluxated Lens

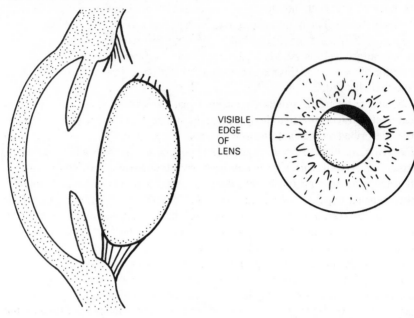

VISIBLE
EDGE
OF
LENS

Figure 17.25: Dislocated Lens

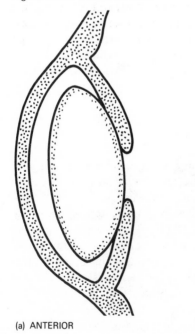

(a) ANTERIOR   (b) POSTERIOR

18 THE VITREOUS

Introduction

Most disorders of the vitreous manifest themselves by the presence of opacities in what is normally an optically transparent structure. Because the vitreous moves like a jelly with each eye movement such opacities also move. By causing a shadow on the retina these opacities appear to the patient as floating black shapes ('floaters') which dance annoyingly in the field of vision. Many vitreous disorders are due primarily to disease of the retina or choroid. However, haemorrhages and exudates clear more slowly from the secondarily involved vitreous than from the diseased retina or choroid because the vitreous is poorly supplied with phagocytes.

Congenital Anomalies

Parts of the hyaloid system of vessels may persist and be visible with the ophthalmoscope. Muscae volitantes ('flitting flies') are tiny floaters which are present in most people but which are often invisible to the examiner. They are probably due to minute hyaloid remnants and are quite harmless. Rarely, the foetal vitreous persists as a dense mass behind the lens (persistent hyperplastic primary vitreous); this is usually first detected in infancy because the pupil appears white (leucocoria).

Vitreous Degenerations

These are common in aged, myopic or diseased eyes.

Asteroid Hyalosis and Synchysis Scintillans

These are names given to white opacities which may be more apparent to the examiner than the patient. The former are white and the latter shiny and glittering.

Liquefaction

Most vitreous degenerations and inflammations are accompanied by liquefaction. This makes opacities become more mobile and noticeable.

Detachment

With age the vitreous commonly becomes detached from the retina and collapses towards the lens. The space created fills with aqueous. The patient may see flashing lights at the time of detachment and afterwards a floater. The latter is due to a shadow cast by the posterior vitreous surface which may be visible with the ophthalmoscope. Vitreous detachment is harmless in itself but may be accompanied by a retinal tear with its own attendant risks.

Exudate

Choroiditis causes an outpouring of inflammatory exudates and cells into the vitreous. The patient complains of blurred vision and floaters; vitreous haze obscures the fundus. Such exudates clear slowly as the condition subsides but repeated attacks may result in a permanently hazy vitreous with poor vision.

Haemorrhage

Vitreous haemorrhage may arise from trauma, a retinal tear, or from retinal new vessels in disorders such as proliferative diabetic retinopathy or following central retinal vein occlusion. With a small haemorrhage the patient complains of floaters but larger haemorrhages completely obscure the retina and cause a profound worsening of vision. These haemorrhages usually clear slowly but often fresh bleeding occurs so that vision progressively deteriorates. It is therefore vital to find the cause of the haemorrhage and institute treatment to prevent further bleeds. If there is no history of trauma, diabetes or venous occlusion and especially if the patient has experienced flashes of light, a retinal tear should be assumed to be present. Such a patient should be admitted for bedrest in hospital; sometimes both eyes are padded to reduce eye movements. With this regimen the haemorrhage may clear sufficiently to allow treatment with either cryotherapy or photocoagulation.

Vitrectomy

Opaque vitreous may be removed in one of two ways. In the 'open sky' technique a disc of cornea is removed and the lens and vitreous extracted piecemeal through this hole; afterwards the disc is sutured in place. In pars plana vitrectomy a special instrument is inserted via the pars plana six millimetres behind the limbus. This instrument simultaneously cuts the vitreous, aspirates it and replaces it with a balanced salt solution. A dense vitreous haemorrhage which has failed to clear spontaneously may be removed in this way. However, improved vision will result only if the previously obscured retina is still functioning and provided this hazardous operation is free from major complications.

19 THE RETINA

The retina is a highly specialised tissue. It is supplied by both retinal and choroidal circulations. Because there is no anastomosis between either the retinal and choroidal vessels or between branches of the retinal vessels themselves, occlusive episodes are followed by retinal hypoxia with profound effects.

The macula itself is free of blood vessels; this is obviously desirable as the contained blood would interfere with light transmission to the cones. However, its avascularity renders it particularly vulnerable to hypoxia, toxins etc., so macular degenerations are common. Unfortunately, lesions of the macula, though minute in size, are crippling in their effects.

Fluorescein Fundus Angiography (FFA)

If fluorescein (20 per cent) is injected into a vein it rapidly appears in the retinal and choroidal blood vessels. For a short time these vessels fluoresce if they are illuminated by blue light and their architecture can be studied. With a suitable filter in the camera, photographs can be taken in rapid sequence to show how first the retinal arteries, then the capillaries and then the veins fill with the dye. Finally, the fluorescein is eliminated from the retinal circulation. The dye in the choroid is usually masked from view by the retinal pigment epithelium.

Normal retinal vessels and the retinal pigment epithelium are impermeable to fluorescein so that the retina itself should not fluoresce. Choroidal vessels, however, are permeable to the dye. Any defects in the retinal pigment epithelial layer allow choroidal fluorescence to show through; these are termed transmission or 'window' defects. Abnormal retinal capillaries leak fluorescein. Thus fluorescein angiography may be used to delineate abnormal retinal vessels (e.g., in tumours) and to identify 'window' defects and leaking retinal vessels in disorders such as diabetic retinopathy and macular degeneration.

Fluorescein angiography is carried out as an out-patient procedure. After dilating the pupils fully, colour photographs are taken of the fundi. Fluorescein is then injected rapidly into an arm vein and black and white photographs are taken through a blue filter in a rapid sequence. Patients often feel sick for a few seconds after the injection. Allergic reactions such as rashes, bronchospasm or cardiovascular collapse may also occur and so appropriate drugs such as chlorpheniramine (Piriton), hydrocortisone and adrenaline must be readily available.

Photocoagulation

Intense light may be directed through the cornea and focused on to the retina to create burns. The instruments commonly used to do this are the Xenon Arc Photocoagulator and the Argon Laser. They may be used to seal retinal holes by creating inflammatory adhesions between the retina and the choroid. Pigment epithelial defects and abnormal vessels may also be sealed. Photocoagulation can be carried out under local anaesthesia on an out-patient basis but admission to hospital and general anaesthesia is sometimes advisable. Full mydriasis is always required. Several sessions are sometimes necessary to complete treatment.

Vascular Disorders

General

Many systemic diseases produce characteristic changes in blood vessels. In the retina, and nowhere else, we can see these changes during life. Thus fundus examination is frequently useful in the diagnosis of diseases such as hypertension, diabetes, sickle cell anaemia, leukaemia, etc. Moreover, these diseases may threaten the patient's eyesight because of the retinal vascular changes they induce. Vascular occlusions, vasculitis and neovascularisation may occur. (See chapter 22.)

Neovascularisation (New Vessel Formation)

Retinal hypoxia, secondary to diabetes, venous occlusions, vasculitis, etc., may stimulate the growth of new blood vessels. (Complete anoxia, following arterial occlusions, rarely cause neovascularisation.) These vessels may grow 'flat' against the retina or 'forward' into the vitreous. They are fragile and liable to leak and bleed. Vessels growing forward from the optic disc are particularly likely to cause vitreous haemorrhages with resultant loss of sight.

Photocoagulation of all the hypoxic retina can be used to prevent further neovascularisation or to encourage existing vessels to regress.

Central Retinal Artery Occlusion (CRAO)

This may arise as a complication of arteriosclerosis, hypertension, diabetes, temporal arteritis, migraine, or treatment with drugs such as oral contraceptives. Occlusion of the artery may be due to spasm of the arterial wall or to an embolus or thrombus obliterating its lumen.

Signs and Symptoms. The patient's vision falls suddenly and painlessly, usually to no perception of light. Some hours afterwards, ophthalmoscopy will reveal a milky white retina due to oedema of the ganglion cell layer. By contrast, the macula appears as a 'cherry red' spot since it has no ganglion cells. The vessels become attenuated. The causative embolus may be seen at the optic disc. Unless the occlusion is relieved, optic atrophy develops and the patient remains blind in that eye.

Treatment. Various manoeuvres, if applied within hours of the event, are occasionally successful in relieving the obstruction. They include rebreathing air in a bag (the raised carbon dioxide level dilates blood vessels), a retrobulbar injection of vasodilator substances such as tolazoline (Priscol) or lowering the intraocular pressure by intravenous acetazolamide and paracentesis of the anterior chamber. Underlying diseases, such as temporal arteritis, must obviously be treated to prevent further vascular accidents.

Central Retinal Vein Occlusion (CRVO)

This may arise as a complication of glaucoma, arteriosclerosis, hypertension, diabetes or blood disorders (e.g., leukaemia). These diseases may cause an occlusion because of pressure on the vein or be due to disease of the vein wall. Alternatively, the occlusion may be the result of stagnation of the blood column.

Signs and Symptoms. The patient's vision falls painlessly. Some vision is usually retained. Ophthalmoscopy reveals dilated veins and numerous haemorrhages scattered throughout the whole fundus.

Complications. New blood vessels commonly develop. If they arise in the retina, vitreous haemorrhages may occur with further loss of vision. New vessels may also arise in the drainage angle provoking thrombotic glaucoma (see chapter 16), usually about three months after the venous occlusion. ('A hundred-day glaucoma'.) This catastrophe often leads to loss of the eye.

Treatment. No treatment is likely to improve vision but any underlying disease that threatens the fellow eye must be treated. Anticoagulants are occasionally given. Destruction of hypoxic retina by photocoagulation may reduce or reverse the formation of new blood vessels which themselves further threaten the patient's eyesight.

Branch Retinal Vein Occlusion

This has a similar aetiology to central retinal vein occlusion. Occlusion of the nasal branches often passes unnoticed by the patient but may be seen with the ophthalmoscope. Temporal branch vein occlusion commonly causes oedema of the macula with some visual disturbance. Treatment is essentially as for central retinal vein occlusion.

Vasculitis

Inflammatory involvement of retinal vessels may be a feature of sarcoidosis, uveitis, and other rarer conditions. Veins are more commonly affected than arteries or capillaries. Examination may show perivascular haemorrhages and sheathing as well as vitreous opacities. Fluorescein angiography may demonstrate leakage from vessels. Vasculitis may completely resolve or lead to obliteration of the vessels with resulting retinal hypoxia or neovascularisation. Systemic steroids and photocoagulation may be required.

Coats' Disease (Retinal Telangiectasis)

This uncommon condition is classically unilateral and affects young males. A mass of white exudate collects between the choroid and retina, probably following a haemorrhage from an area of retinal telangiectasia which is usually present. As the exudate increases, the patient may develop a squint, leucocoria and finally a blind disorganised eye. Enucleation may be required.

Inflammatory Disorders — Toxoplasmosis

This is an infection with the protozoan parasite *Toxoplasma gondii.*

Primary Infection

This is usually acquired by eating contaminated meat. The patient suffers a mild illness with a fever and a rash. Antibodies develop and the patient recovers unharmed.

Secondary Infection

If a pregnant woman acquires toxoplasmosis the organisms simultaneously invade the fetus and are preserved in cysts immune to attack from antibodies. Shortly before or after birth these cysts rupture releasing organisms which cause a severe infection in the baby with retino-choroiditis and encephalitis. Varying degrees of brain damage and retinal scarring result. Encysted organisms may then persist in the eye until adulthood.

Infection becomes apparent when encysted organisms are released in an adult who had the primary infection in fetal life. It is the commonest form of acute chorio-retinitis occurring in England.

Signs and Symptoms. Typically the patient complains of blurred vision because the vitreous becomes invaded with inflammatory cells and exudate. If the macula is involved, the visual loss is profound. Vitreous opacities can be seen with the ophthalmoscope. They may obscure the involved part of the retina which becomes white. When the inflammation subsides, the vitreous clears to reveal a pigmented chorio-retinal scar. This is always adjacent to other scars from past (possibly intrauterine) infection.

Investigation. Toxoplasma antibody levels may be measured by the *Toxo-*

plasma dye test. The test is often not helpful since most adults have antibodies arising from undiagnosed primary infection and acute chorio-retinitis is often not accompanied by increased antibody production. However, the absence of antibodies does exclude toxoplasmosis. An increasing level of titres on serial testing denotes active infection.

Treatment. Pyrimethamine (Daraprim) and sulphonamides will kill free organisms but not encysted forms so that recurrences are not prevented. These drugs may cause agranulocytosis so they are rarely prescribed. Acute chorio-retinitis is often treated with systemic steroids. These reduce intraocular inflammation and minimise scarring.

Note. Toxoplasmosis is only infective in the primary stage. Pregnant women should obviously avoid patients with primary infection but unfortunately the infection is rarely diagnosed at this stage. Patients with acute chorio-retinitis are not infective and a pregnant woman with chorio-retinitis need not fear that her baby will be harmed by infection, although the fetus may be harmed by systemic steroids.

Degenerations — Retinitis Pigmentosa

This is a chronic progressive degeneration of the retina of unknown cause. It is most often inherited as an autosomal recessive disease. It affects both eyes and commonly becomes apparent in late childhood.

Signs and Symptoms

The patient, who usually has affected relatives, notices increasing difficulty seeing in the dark due to degeneration of the rods. The visual fields become constricted. Initially a ring scotoma develops; then there is progressive loss of the peripheral field until there is only tunnel vision, albeit with good visual acuity. Finally, even the central vision is affected as the cones, too, degenerate and the patient often becomes totally blind (Figure 19.1). Fundus examination reveals a characteristic picture with clumps of pigment cells, narrowed arterioles and optic atrophy.

Associated Diseases

Some patients with retinitis pigmentosa also have neurological abnormalities, defects of the skeletal system, mental deficiency and other ocular abnormalities — particularly cataracts.

Treatment

There is no known cure for this disease. Patients can be helped by using low vision aids and by retraining for occupations which do not require sight. Genetic

Figure 19.1: Field in Retinitis Pigmentosa

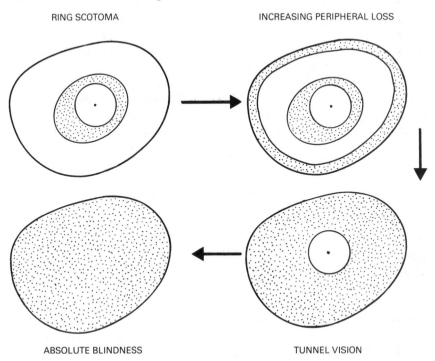

RING SCOTOMA   INCREASING PERIPHERAL LOSS

ABSOLUTE BLINDNESS   TUNNEL VISION

counselling should reduce the number of potentially affected individuals that are born. Patients' relatives should be examined by ophthalmoscopy, field testing and electrical tests (ERG, EOG) so that early cases can be identified and offered advice about their future needs.

Trauma (see chapter 23)

Congenital and Developmental Abnormalities

Myelinated Nerve Fibres

A relatively common abnormality is the presence of a white fluffy patch in the retina usually near the optic disc due to myelination of the nerve fibre layer. A corresponding field defect may be elicited since myelin is opaque and may prevent light reaching the rods and cones. Usually the patient is not inconvenienced and the abnormality is only elicited during routine ophthalmoscopy.

Retrolental Fibroplasia (Retinopathy of Prematurity)

This disease was rife in the 1940s and at its peak rendered 20 to 30 per cent of premature babies blind. Its precise cause is not yet known. An abnormally high concentration of oxygen reaching the immature retina appears to be contributory. Retinal vascularisation is not complete until 38 weeks gestation. Before this time excess oxygen constricts immature capillaries. On withdrawal of oxygen new capillaries proliferate. They may grow into the vitreous and promote fibrosis: as a result traction detachments of the retina occur. Ultimately a white retrolental mass of fibrous tissue and detached retina may result. Mild cases resolve spontaneously. Severe cases tend to deteriorate further in later life. Theoretically the disorder could be prevented by ensuring that the arterial oxygen concentration of premature babies is kept between 60 to 90 mmHg. Monitoring the oxygen concentration in the incubator itself is no guarantee of safety. In practice these criteria may be hard to fulfill so, unfortunately, almost certainly, cases will continue to occur.

Tumours — Retinoblastoma

This is the commonest primary intraocular tumour apart from malignant melanoma. Some cases are inherited as an autosomal dominant disorder. It is bilateral in 20 to 30 per cent of cases. It usually occurs within the first few years of life. The tumour arises within the retina but later fills the eyeball and extends to extraocular tissues. Spread commonly occurs via the optic nerve and cerebrospinal fluid. Blood borne metastases also occur.

Signs and Symptoms

The child may present with a squint because the vision of the affected eye is poor. Leucocoria may be present. Later the eye may be red, painful and glaucomatous because the tumour has obstructed the outflow of aqueous. In advanced cases there is proptosis and involvement of the periorbital tissues. The tumour is likely to be fatal if extraocular spread has occurred.

Investigation

A suspected case should be examined under general anaesthesia as soon as possible. Both eyes are examined under full mydriasis for sometimes both eyes are affected. Several Consultants may be asked to give their opinion, particularly if enucleation is contemplated.

Treatment

Small tumours can be treated by external cobalt irradiation or by the application of a radioactive cobalt plaque to the eye. Enucleation is required if the optic nerve is thought to be involved or if the eye is glaucomatous. Photocoagulation or cryotherapy may be used for recurrences or for small tumours in the fellow eye. Regular follow-up examinations are necessary so that recurrences can be diagnosed and treated whilst they are small. The survival rate in the United Kingdom is about 85 per cent.

Genetic Counselling

It is usually possible to estimate the risk of a retinoblastoma arising in the relatives of an affected individual. The risk is highest if the tumour is bilateral or if there are affected relatives. Children at risk should be examined under anaesthesia regularly so that the tumours may be detected and treated at an early stage.

Phakomata

These are congenital tumours of the retina and central nervous system. They are multiple and often familial. The effects of them may not be apparent until early adulthood. They are usually accompanied by characteristic skin blemishes. Four types of phakomata are recognised as occurring in distinctive syndromes as follows.

Von Recklinghausen's Disease (Neurofibromatosis)

This is the commonest type of phakomata. It is characterised by peripheral nerve tumours, which can be felt under the skin, and brown skin lesions called 'café-au-lait' spots. In addition to these less serious manifestations, an optic nerve glioma or an acoustic neuroma may develop. The former may blind and the latter may kill the patient.

The Sturge-Weber Syndrome

Vascular tumours occur in the skin, meninges and retina. Classically the patient has an unsightly red area on one side of his face (a port wine stain). The eye on the affected side may have dilated conjunctival vessels and be glaucomatous.

Tuberose Sclerosis

This is characterised by waxy lesions in the skin (adenoma sebaceum), 'mulberry' tumours in the retina, and tumours in the brain.

The Von Hippel-Lindau Syndrome

There are vascular tumours in the retina and in the cerebellum. Retinal and vitreous haemorrhages are possible complications.

Macular Disease

Senile Macular Degeneration (SMD)

This is one of the commonest causes of blindness in the United Kingdom. Both eyes are usually affected, though often asymmetrically.

Signs and Symtoms. There is gradual painless loss of central vision as the macula becomes degenerate. The peripheral retina is unaffected so that blindness is never absolute and a wide visual field is retained. Occasionally a macular haemorrhage occurs and the patient's vision suddenly worsens. Ophthalmoscopy may reveal colloid bodies (white spots), abnormal pigmentation, oedema and haemorrhage at the macula; choroidal vessels may be visible through the degenerate retina. Disciform macular degeneration is a severe form in which there is gross macular disruption with oedema and haemorrhage; the visual acuity is markedly reduced.

Treatment. Patients should be re-assured that their sight will never be completely lost. They may be helped by using a low vision aid and also by their being entered on the register as being either Partially Sighted or Blind (chapter 25). Laser photocoagulation can sometimes be used to arrest the condition or to prevent visual loss in the fellow eye.

Heredo-macular Degeneration

Macular degeneration occasionally occurs in younger people when it is commonly hereditary. Other macular and cerebral defects may be present.

Central Serous Retinopathy

This condition usually affects young men who complain of blurred vision in one eye. Things viewed with the affected eye may appear darker and look smaller (micropsia). Fundus examination reveals oedema of the macula and angiography shows a leaking vessel in association with a break in Bruch's membrane. The condition usually resolves completely without treatment but recurrences are common. Photocoagulation, to seal the break, is usually reserved for recurrent cases.

Oedema Following Trauma

Macular oedema may complicate blunt injuries to the eye and solar burns, incurred when viewing an eclipse of the sun without adequate protection of the eye (chapter 23).

Macular Damage Due to Drugs

Chloroquine, used in the treatment of malaria and rheumatoid arthritis, may cause macular damage if the dose exceeds one hundred grams in one year. The patient's vision deteriorates and the macula shows abnormal pigmented rings (Bull's eye maculopathy). Patients on long-term chloroquine should have regular eye checks and report immediately if their vision deteriorates. Unfortunately, the macular damage is usually irreversible.

Retinal Detachment

A retinal detachment occurs when the neuro-retina separates from the underlying pigment layer. These two layers come together in intrauterine life when the optic cup invaginates (Figure 19.2), but they can be easily stripped apart except at the ora serrata. Detachments are most often due to a hole in the neuroretina which allows fluid vitreous to track between the two layers and separate them; the collection of fluid is then termed subretinal fluid (SRF). However, detachments do occur without holes in conditions in which fluid is secreted by either the retina or the choroid.

Retinal Holes

These usually arise in the thin peripheral retina between the equator and the ora serrata. They may be single or multiple, round or 'U' shaped (horseshoe) and often occur in degenerate or damaged retina. A dialysis, or disinsertion, is a large tear at the ora serrata. The lifted edges of horseshoe tears and dialyses indicate traction on the retina by vitreous strands; a detachment is the likely sequel to such tears unless they are promptly sealed. This may be achieved by photocoagulation or cryotherapy with or without scleral indentation, under local or general anaesthesia. The treatment of retinal holes is easier, quicker and more successful than the treatment of retinal detachments.

Retinal Detachment Due to Holes in the Retina

High myopia, previous cataract extraction (especially if vitreous loss has occurred), a family history of detachment or severe ocular trauma all predispose to this kind of detachment.

Signs and Symptoms. An observant patient may notice flashes of light when the retinal tear occurs, followed by floaters as blood from the torn retina enters the

Figure 19.2: Invagination of the Optic Vesicle

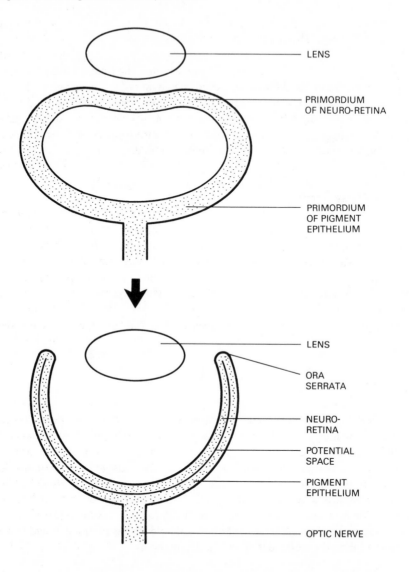

vitreous. After a variable interval of time, the detachment develops and is accompanied by loss of vision because the neuro-retina cannot function unless it is in contact with the pigment epithelium. Initially there is only a field defect; this will be in the upper field of vision if the inferior part of the retina is detached and vice versa. The patient may complain of a 'curtain' falling over his vision. Later, when the macula detaches, a profound drop in visual acuity occurs. Untreated, the detachment often becomes total; the vision falls to no perception of light and the eye may shrink. Occasionally a detachment arrests spontaneously.

Classically, examination demonstrates a field defect and ophthalmoscopy reveals the detached retina as a dark billowing area with red choroid showing through the hole. However, appearances vary and the diagnosis is sometimes difficult.

Management. Once a detachment has occurred the immediate aim must be to prevent it extending, particularly if the macula is uninvolved. Bed rest in hospital is usually advised. Sometimes eye movements are discouraged by covering both eyes or by the use of pin-hole spectacles. The patient is positioned so that the causative hole is lowermost; thus patients with inferior detachments are nursed sitting up. Sometimes subretinal fluid resolves during bed rest. This renders operation easier.

Meanwhile, the retina is repeatedly and thoroughly examined after maximum mydriasis often using the three mirror contact lens as well as both the direct and indirect ophthalmoscopes. The surgeon may make a drawing of the detachment, the holes and important retinal landmarks to assist him at operation. The fellow eye should be examined under mydriasis so that any retinal holes detected can be treated prophylactically.

Surgery. The aim of surgery is to flatten the detached neuro-retina against the pigment epithelium so preventing further extension of the detachment and restoring vision. Re-attachment is accompanied by restoration of the visual field but the visual acuity may not improve if the macula is detached. Closure of all retinal holes is vital to prevent re-accumulation of sub-retinal fluid. The neural and pigment layers of the retina are approximated by indenting the sclera, and perhaps by releasing sub-retinal fluid or expanding the vitreous volume. These procedures counteract vitreous traction (see Figure 19.3). Each operation must be tailor-made for the particular patient.

The operation is usually carried out under general anaesthesia. Full mydriasis is necessary so that the surgeon has a good view of the retina. The sclera overlying the detachment is exposed by incising the conjunctiva and by retracting the extraocular muscles. The holes are localised by indirect ophthalmoscopy, with indentation, and their position marked on the overlying sclera. The holes are usually sealed by monitored cryotherapy which creates an inflammatory adhesion between the retina and the choroid.

Scleral indentation may be achieved by scleral resection, by sewing a silastic plomb to the sclera, by inserting fascia lata into a pocket created within the scleral layers, or by sewing a silicone band around the globe (encirclement). The indentation should overlie the holes. Incising the sclera and choroid over the detachment to allow sub-retinal fluid to drain out is useful in extensive detachments but may be complicated by haemorrhage or intraocular infection. Sub-retinal fluid may also be drained through a needle within the eye. Expansion of

Figure 19.3: Methods of Approximating Retinal Layers

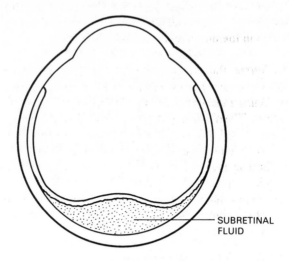

SUBRETINAL
FLUID

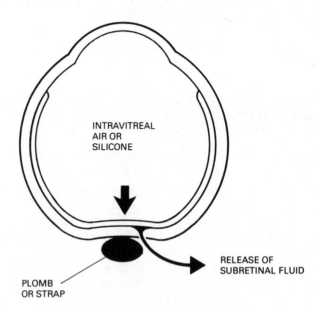

INTRAVITREAL
AIR OR
SILICONE

RELEASE OF
SUBRETINAL FLUID

PLOMB
OR STRAP

the vitreous by intravitreal injection of air or silicone carries similar risks. Before concluding the operation the surgeon examines the fundus closely to ensure that the indentation is correctly sited and that the central retinal artery has not been occluded by a rise in the intraocular pressure.

Post-operative Course. Patients may require analgesia, especially after encircling operations. Excessive pain may be due to infection or to raised intraocular pressure. Once ophthalmoscopy shows that the retina has flattened the patient is gradually mobilised. The return to normal activities should be gradual and heavy lifting should be avoided. Patients are warned to report fresh episodes of 'flashes' and 'floaters' and to check that their visual fields remain full. Follow-up examinations of both eyes are advisable so that fresh retinal holes can be detected and treated before detachment occurs.

If the retina does not flatten a second operation may be advised. However, operations on long-standing detachments or detachments with much vitreous traction are unlikely to succeed.

Retinal Detachment Without Holes

Sub-retinal fluid may be formed in inflammatory conditions e.g., scleritis and choroiditis or retinal vascular disorders e.g., toxaemia of pregnancy. Systemic steroids may be beneficial in inflammatory conditions. Fluid may also accompany a malignant melanoma of the choroid.

Retinoschisis

This is a split within the neuro-retina and may resemble a detachment. It is often bilateral and symptomless. Operation is unnecessary unless the schisis begins to encroach on the macula or a true detachment supervenes.

THE OPTIC NERVE AND CENTRAL NERVOUS SYSTEM

The Optic Nerve

The optic nerve differs from all other nerves in that it is part of the central nervous system and it is surrounded by meninges and the subarachnoid space over its entire length. Because of these factors and because of its close proximity to the pituitary gland and the internal carotid arteries, it is involved in many conditions affecting the brain. The appearance of the optic disc may be a useful pointer to many of these diseases.

Optic Neuritis: Papillitis and Retrobulbar Neuritis

Patients with inflammation of the optic nerve (optic neuritis) may go on to develop signs of multiple sclerosis after a variable interval of time. Occasionally the neuritis is associated with a viral infection (*Herpes zoster*) or infection of the ethmoid air cells. Sometimes the cause is not determined.

Signs and Symptoms

Young women are most often affected. There is a sudden onset of pain in the affected eye; this is increased by movement of the eye. The vision falls rapidly and a dense central scotoma develops. On examination the pupils react poorly to a light shone on the affected eye (afferent pupil defect — see p.196). The globe may be tender.

If the inflammation occurs at the optic nerve head, the optic disc (papilla) appears swollen and there may be haemorrhages on it. This is sometimes called papillitis. If the inflammation affects that part of the optic nerve some way behind the globe, the optic disc appears quite normal and the condition is known as retrobulbar neuritis. Sometimes the fellow optic nerve is affected shortly after the first. The attack begins to resolve within a few days. The pain subsides and the patient's vision improves. However, the optic disc may become pale after a few weeks (i.e., optic atrophy develops). Patients sometimes complain that the quality of their vision remains impaired even when the acuity has recovered to 6/6 on the Snellen Chart.

Treatment

Unless an underlying cause (e.g., sinusitis) can be found, there is no specific treatment. Systemic steroids or ACTH may be given to shorten the time during which the patient's vision is impaired. This is particularly desirable if both eyes are affected. Unfortunately, this treatment does not affect the eventual visual outcome.

Patients sometimes have another attack of neuritis months or years later.

Ischaemic Optic Neuropathy

The optic nerve head, although pierced by the central retinal artery, is nourished by the posterior ciliary arteries. A sudden occlusion of these arteries may arise in elderly patients with giant cell arteritis or generalised arteriosclerosis. There is a sudden and marked deterioration in vision and the optic disc becomes swollen and pale due to ischaemia.

An ESR estimation should always be performed as patients with giant cell arteritis must be given large doses of systemic steroids to prevent a similar occlusion in the other eye. Such treatment rarely benefits the ischaemic eye.

Papilloedema

Papillitis means swelling of the optic disc due to inflammation. Papilloedema means swelling of the optic nerve without inflammation and is usually due to raised intracranial pressure or malignant hypertension.

Raised intracranial pressure is transmitted to the subarachnoid space around the optic nerve. Increased pressure within the optic nerve obstructs axoplasmic transport and venous blood flow. Thus the swelling of papilloedema is thought to consist of accumulated axoplasm and transudate from veins.

Papilloedema is often the earliest objective evidence of raised intracranial pressure due to a cerebral tumour. Hence, fundus examination is a vital part of the examination of patients suspected of having such a tumour.

Signs and Symptoms

Papilloedema is detected with the ophthalmoscope as a swelling of the optic nerve head. The disc margin becomes blurred and the disc itself becomes more pink. The vessels lying on the disc become engorged and a few flame-shaped haemorrhages may appear around the edge of the disc. Binocular methods of ophthalmoscopy and stereophotographs are particularly useful in detecting early cases. Fluorescein angiography may help to distinguish cases of papilloedema from the apparently elevated discs of those who are hypermetropic (pseudo-papilloedema).

The vision is normal in early cases of papilloedema. Later it drops dramatically and optic atrophy develops. Papilloedema will regress once the intracranial pressure is relieved but this should be done speedily to prevent the development of optic atrophy.

Optic Atrophy

This is a condition in which the optic nerve fibres die and the optic nerve diminishes in size. If fibres from the macula are affected the visual acuity will fall. If fibres from the retinal periphery are affected then there will be loss of visual field. Ultimately the patient's vision may fall to no perception of light. The optic disc becomes very pale. The pupils will react poorly or not at all when a light is shone on the affected eye.

Causes

Optic atrophy may result from damage to the nerve fibres anywhere along their course from the ganglion cells in the retina to their termination in the lateral geniculate body (Figure 20.1).

Conditions such as retinitis pigmentosa and central retinal artery occlusion cause damage to the nerve fibres on their way to the disc and are said to cause ascending optic atrophy. Other conditions such as tumours and aneurysms damage fibres beyond the disc and are said to cause descending optic atrophy. In glaucoma, papilloedema and papillitis the lesion is at the disc itself. In some conditions, e.g., toxic amblyopia and hereditary optic atrophy, the site of the lesion is unknown.

The treatment of optic atrophy is that of the cause. The visual loss is usually irreversible but further deterioration may be prevented.

Vascular Causes of Optic Atrophy

Ischaemia, following central retinal artery occlusion or ischaemic optic neuropathy, is one of the commonest causes of optic atrophy. It usually affects the elderly.

Glaucoma

Glaucoma, particularly chronic open-angle glaucoma, is another common cause of optic atrophy but here the disc pallor is accompanied by characteristic cupping of the nerve head because the supporting tissue, as well as the nerve fibres, is lost.

Tumours

Tumours are an important cause of optic atrophy. The visual loss is gradual and painless. The tumour may arise within the nerve itself or press on the nerve from without.

Optic Nerve Glioma. This is a tumour that arises within the optic nerve, often in young people. It may complicate neuro-fibromatosis. The swollen nerve commonly causes proptosis and enlargement of the optic foramen. Extension into the chiasm or brain may occur with fatal results.

Figure 20.1: Causes of Optic Atrophy

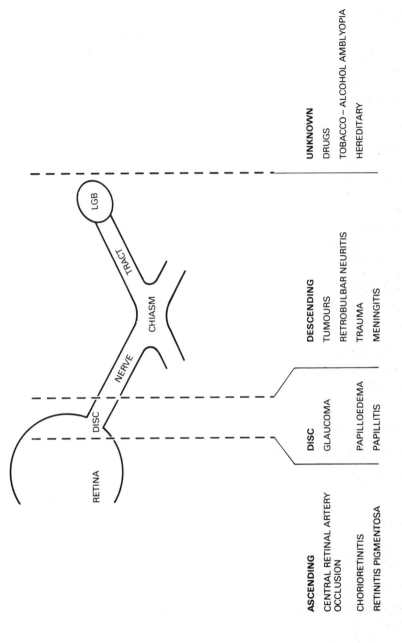

RETINA

DISC

NERVE

TRACT

CHIASM

LGB

ASCENDING

CENTRAL RETINAL ARTERY OCCLUSION

CHORIORETINITIS

RETINITIS PIGMENTOSA

DISC

GLAUCOMA

PAPILLOEDEMA

PAPILLITIS

DESCENDING

TUMOURS

RETROBULBAR NEURITIS

TRAUMA

MENINGITIS

UNKNOWN

DRUGS

TOBACCO – ALCOHOL AMBLYOPIA

HEREDITARY

Meningioma. These tumours may arise within the orbit (from the optic nerve sheath) or within the skull. They are benign tumours and can sometimes be removed surgically.

Pituitary Tumours. Pituitary tumours that enlarge forward as well as upwards may press on the optic nerve and cause optic atrophy. It is usually the non-hormone secreting tumours in adults and craniopharyngiomas in children that do this. These tumours can be successfully treated by operation or irradiation so that early diagnosis is imperative.

Demyelination

An episode of retrobulbar neuritis may be followed by optic atrophy.

Trauma

Severe head injuries are sometimes followed by optic atrophy because the blood supply to the optic nerve has been damaged either by bony splinters or by pressure from oedematous tissues. Loss of vision is instantaneous but often several weeks elapse before the disc becomes pale.

Meningitis

Bacterial or tuberculous meningitis may be followed by optic atrophy.

Drugs

Drugs such as ethambutol (used in the treatment of tuberculosis) may cause optic atrophy. The patient's vision occasionally improves if these drugs are withdrawn as soon as a deterioration is noted.

Tobacco-Alcohol Amblyopia

Various toxins and vitamin deficiences may cause optic atrophy. Tobacco-alcohol amblyopia is the only common condition in this group encountered in this country. It occurs in individuals who smoke and drink heavily and who eat a poor diet. The vision may improve if the patient can be persuaded to give up both tobacco and alcohol. Large doses of Vitamin B_{12} given intramuscularly (usually as hydroxy-cobalamin), may be beneficial.

The Optic Chiasm

The chiasm contains the nerve fibres passing from the optic nerves to the optic tracts. It lies above and in front of the pituitary gland and inside the circle of Willis (see chapter 2). Pituitary tumours enlarging upwards and forwards (as they usually do) damage the central part of the chiasm which contains the crossing fibres from the nasal halves of the retinae. If these nasal fibres are damaged the temporal field of vision is lost in both eyes. This is called a bitemporal

Figure 20.2: Lesions at the Optic Chiasm. Bitemporal Hemianopia

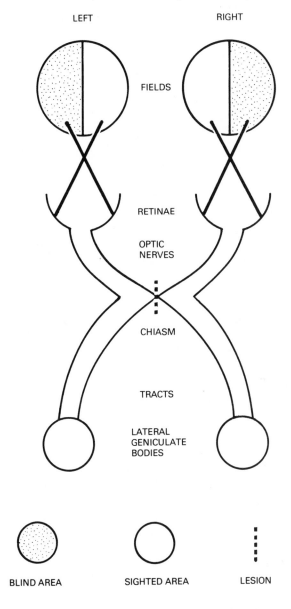

hemianopia and is almost diagnostic of a pituitary tumour. Aneurysms occasionally produce a similar field loss (Figure 20.2).

The Optic Radiation

The optic radiation contains fibres passing from the lateral geniculate body to the occipital cortex. The right optic radiation carries impulses from the left halves of the visual fields and vice versa (see chapter 2).

The radiation is supplied by branches of the middle cerebral artery which arises from the internal carotid artery. Sudden occlusion of the middle cerebral artery or internal carotid artery is a relatively common form of cerebro-vascular accident ('stroke'). A left-sided occlusion leads to loss of the right halves of the visual fields causing a right homonymous hemianopia (Figure 20.3). The patient may have weakness of his right arm and right leg. (The pyramidal fibres cross the midline lower down.) An homonymous hemianopia leads to difficulty with reading and getting about. No treatment will improve the vision but an explanation may help the patient to cope with his disability. The patient should be taught to turn his head towards the side of the hemianopia so as to scan on that side.

An homonymous hemianopia may also be caused by a tumour in the parietal lobe.

The Occipital Cortex

The right occipital cortex receives impulses from the left halves of the visual fields and vice versa. Thus damage to the right occipital cortex by a tumour, trauma or a vascular accident will result in a left homonymous hemianopia.

The tip of the occipital lobe is concerned with macular vision, so it is possible for a blow on the back of the head to result in the loss of central vision while the peripheral vision is retained. 'Cortical blindness' means that a patient is blind from bilateral occipital cortex lesions. The pupils will still react to light (see chapter 2). Strangely, such patients often deny that they are blind.

Cerebro-vascular Accidents and Transient Ischaemic Attacks

The internal carotid arteries and the vertebro-basilar system are commonly occluded by atheroma or by emboli from diseased heart valves. Permanent occlusions result in cerebro-vascular accidents ('strokes'). Temporary occlusions cause episodes of cerebral dysfunction lasting a few minutes before resolving completely. These are termed transient ischaemic attacks (TIAs).

If the right internal carotid artery is temporarily occluded the patient may

Figure 20.3: Lesion of the Left Optic Radiation. Right Homonymous Hemianopia

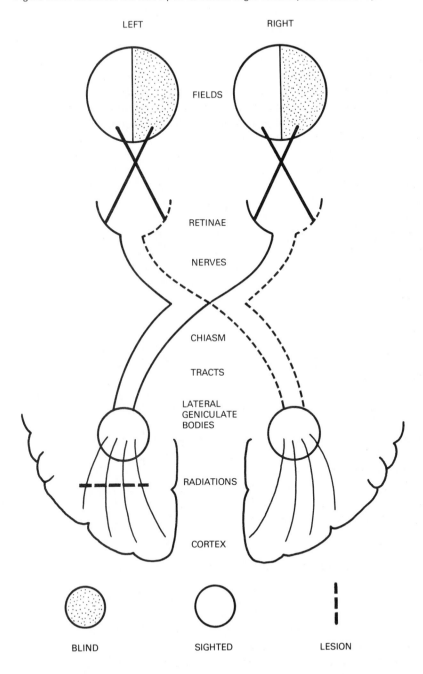

LEFT   RIGHT

FIELDS

RETINAE

NERVES

CHIASM

TRACTS

LATERAL
GENICULATE
BODIES

RADIATIONS

CORTEX

BLIND   SIGHTED   LESION

complain of loss of vision of the right eye lasting a few minutes. This is because the internal carotid artery (through branches of the ophthalmic artery) supplies the optic nerve and retina. There may be other signs and symptoms such as hemiplegia and parasthesiae.

If the vertebro-basilar system is affected the patient may complain of transient hemianopias because the optic radiations are supplied by these arteries. There may be other signs and symptoms such as vertigo and nystagmus.

Transient ischaemic attacks may be the forerunners of a completed stroke, so such patients should be investigated for treatable medical conditions.

Aneurysms

Saccular aneurysms are balloon-shaped out-pouchings from an artery. They are quite common on the arteries of the circle of Willis. Part of the internal carotid artery may become dilated into a fusiform aneurysm in an arteriosclerotic individual (Figure 20.4).

Figure 20.4: Types of Aneurysm

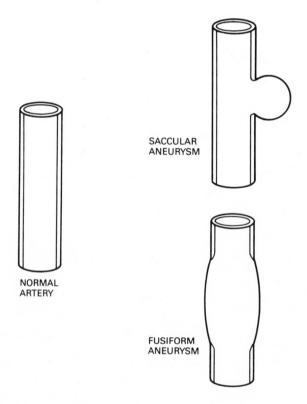

SACCULAR
ANEURYSM

NORMAL
ARTERY

FUSIFORM
ANEURYSM

Aneurysms may cause problems, first, by exerting pressure on adjacent structures as they enlarge. Thus cranial nerve palsies may be due to an aneurysm. Depending on the nerve affected the patient may complain of diplopia or ptosis (see chapters 10 and 21). Pain is usual because the wall of the aneurysm contains nerve fibres which are stretched as the aneurysm bulges.

Secondly, weakened walls of aneurysms may rupture with dramatic consequences. The rupture may be into the brain, into the cerebro-spinal fluid, causing a subarachnoid haemorrhage, or into the cavernous sinus, resulting in a carotico-cavernous fistula.

Carotico-cavernous Fistula

This arises when the internal carotid artery ruptures within the cavernous sinus either because of trauma or because an aneurysmal dilatation finally gives way (Figure 20.5).

Blood under high pressure flows into the cavernous sinus and so through the ophthalmic veins into the orbit. This causes proptosis and the eye may pulsate. The pressure within the orbit damages the optic nerve and the nerves to extraocular muscles so there may be poor vision and diplopia. Glaucoma adds to the pain and visual loss.

Figure 20.5: Carotico-cavernous Fistula

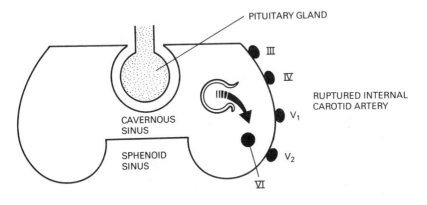

The Pupils

Many conditions affect the size and shape of the pupils. (The pupil reflexes and the factors that influence the pupils in health are considered in chapter 2.) Many diseases of the eye and central nervous system also cause pupil abnormalities. A nurse may be asked to examine the pupils of ophthalmic patients in the post-operative period and of patients undergoing neurological observation. She should record accurately the size and shape of the pupils, whether the two pupils are equal in size and whether there is a brisk reaction to a light directed in each eye in turn. She must also know how to dilate and constrict pupils with drops.

Conditions Causing Dilated Pupil(s) (Mydriasis)

Abnormal mydriasis may be due to a defect in sensory input to the eyes (afferent defect); to a defect in the parasympathetic input to the eye via the third cranial nerve (efferent defect); to an excess input via the sympathetic nerves; or to drugs. In general, parasympathetic lesions have the greatest effect.

Afferent Pupil Defect (Figure 20.6a)

If the retina or optic nerve of, for instance, the left eye is severely damaged (e.g., by trauma or inflammation) the left pupil will not react when a light is shone into the left eye. This is because no impulses are transmitted to the brain. Thus there is no direct light reflex. Because the brain is not stimulated, the right pupil does not react — i.e., there is no consensual light reflex. However, provided there is no other abnormality, when the light is shone in the right eye, the right pupil constricts (because the direct response is intact) and the left pupil also constricts (because the consensual light reflex is intact). These pupil reactions show that it is the pathway to the brain on the left that is at fault and that the patient has a left afferent (towards) pupil defect. The afferent pathway on the right is intact. The efferent (away from) pathways on both sides are intact.

In many cases the damage to the retina or nerve is such that some impulses, rather than none at all, reach the brain. In these instances a relative, rather than an absolute, afferent pupil defect results. In the above example the left pupil, rather than being completely inactive on direct illumination of the left eye, would constrict to some extent.

Efferent Pupil Defect (Figure 20.6b)

Damage to the nucleus of the third cranial (oculomotor) nerve by a tumour or by infarction of the brain stem will cause a dilated, non-reactive pupil on that side. Damage to the third nerve in the skull or orbit by trauma, aneurysm or tumour will have a similar effect.

Haemorrhage within the skull after a head injury may cause a dilated pupil, because the resulting haematoma pushes the brain downwards, crushing the third nerve against the tentorium; this is why the pupil size and pupil reactions are examined regularly after a head injury (neurological observation). Sudden dilatation of one pupil must be reported immediately so that the surgeon can operate to evacuate the haematoma straight away.

Holmes-Adie Pupil

This is a dilated pupil which reacts to accommodation but not to light. It is due to an abnormality in the ciliary ganglion. A Holmes-Adie pupil will constrict after the instillation of 2.5 per cent methacholine drops. A 10 per cent solution is required to cause constriction of the normal pupil.

Acute Glaucoma

Raised intraocular pressure causes the pupil to become semi-dilated because the endings of the ciliary nerves in the iris are damaged.

Traumatic Mydriasis

Blunt trauma may also damage the ciliary nerve endings and cause a dilated pupil. The mydriasis may be permanent.

Cardiac Arrest

Bilaterally dilated pupils are an important sign of cardiac arrest.

Drugs

Sympathomimetic drugs (adrenaline, phenylephrine) dilate the pupils. Anticholinergic drugs (atropine, cyclopentolate, homatropine) are even stronger mydriatics. Local administration of these drugs as drops, ointment or subconjunctival injection usually produces a more profound effect on the pupil than their systemic administration.

Conditions Causing Constricted Pupils (Miosis)

Abnormal miosis may be due to a defect in the sympathetic pathways to the eye, to excess parasympathetic input or to drugs. In general, parasympathetic excess produces the greatest miosis.

Horner's Syndrome

This is due to a defect in the sympathetic pathways causing miosis, ptosis and loss of facial sweating. Damage to the sympathetic pathways anywhere in the head, neck or upper chest may cause this. The commoner causes are syringomyelia and brain stem infarction, trauma of the neck and carcinoma of the lung.

Argyll-Robertson Pupil

This is a small irregular pupil which reacts to accommodation but not to light. It is due to tertiary syphilis. The lesion is thought to be in the brain stem but how it causes the pupillary abnormality is uncertain.

Figure 20.6a. Afferent Pupil Defect

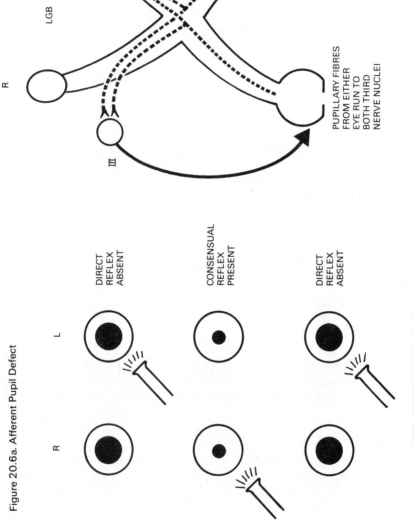

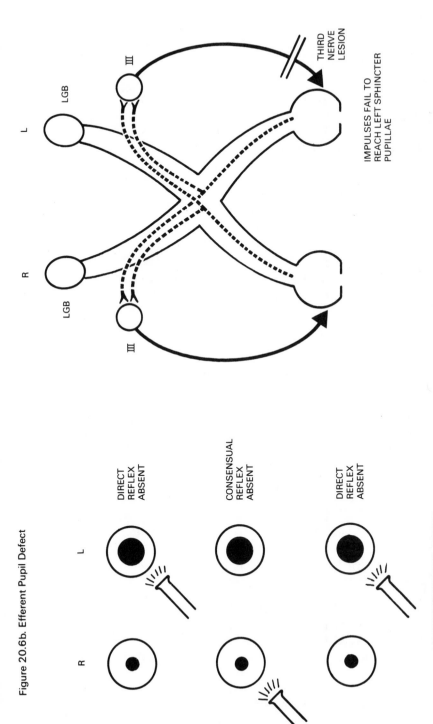

Figure 20.6b. Efferent Pupil Defect

Acute Iritis

This causes constriction of the pupil, usually accompanied by the formation of posterior synechiae.

Drugs

Cholinergic drugs (acetylcholine, pilocarpine) and anticholinesterase inhibitors (physostigmine, ecothiopate iodide) constrict the pupils. In ophthalmic practice, these are used only locally. Some drugs taken systemically constrict the pupils; morphine for instance causes miosis.

Nystagmus

Nystagmus is an involuntary to-and-fro movement of the eyes. Normal individuals have nystagmus when watching stationary objects from a moving vehicle; this is called 'railroad' or optokinetic nystagmus (see below).

Nystagmus may denote a disorder of the eyes or the neuromuscular mechanisms that control eye movements. The former causes pendular nystagmus; the latter causes jerk nystagmus.

Pendular Nystagmus

Here the oscillations are regular and from side to side like a pendulum. It may be due to conditions that have reduced the visual acuity from an early age, such as congenital cataract, macular disease or albinism. It may also be seen in miners who work constantly in poor illumination. Some children with nystagmus have no obvious cataract or macular disease. Their distance vision is usually poor but their reading vision may be quite good, for the nystagmus lessens on near fixation so that normal schooling is possible.

Jerk Nystagmus

Here there is a slow drift of the eyes away from fixation and a quick jerk back. It is the slow drift that is abnormal; the jerk, though more obvious, is a corrective movement. The basic abnormality is a weakness in controlling the direction of gaze, whether this is a voluntary movement or part of a postural reflex (see chapter 2).

The lesion may be in the extraocular muscles, their nerves, the brain stem, cerebellum or inner ear. Multiple sclerosis, brain stem infarction and drugs (e.g., Epanutin) are some common causes.

Jerk nystagmus may be horizontal, vertical or rotary and may be seen only in certain positions of gaze.

The presence of jerk nystagmus and its characteristics may be important diagnostic clues to a neurological abnormality.

Jerk nystagmus does not usually decrease the visual acuity but it may cause the sensation of the environment moving about.

Optokinetic Nystagmus

This a form of jerk nystagmus. It can be produced in normal people by rotating in front of their eyes a drum painted with stripes, provided that the stripes are not too narrow to be seen. An estimate of the visual acuity may be gained by rotating a succession of drums with progressively finer stripes until the patient no longer exhibits nystagmus. The Catford Drum uses this principle but it has spots of graded size instead of stripes.

Cerebral Tumours

Many brain tumours affect the eye. Papilloedema and sixth nerve palsies may arise because of raised intracranial pressure whatever the situation of the tumour. Other signs help to localise the tumour. Optic atrophy may be due to pressure from a frontal lobe tumour. An homonymous hemianopia may be caused by a parietal lobe tumour. Cortical blindness may be due to an occipital lobe tumour. Nystagmus may be a sign of a cerebellar tumour and ophthalmoplegia of a brain stem tumour.

Migraine

This is a severe unilateral headache often accompanied by nausea and vomiting. It often runs in families and is commonest in young adults. The headache may be preceded by an 'aura' lasting a few minutes; the patient may see shimmering zig-zag lines, or he may experience dimming of vision or a hemianopia. Sometimes the headache is accompanied by ophthalmoplegia; usually the third nerve is affected. Migraine is thought to be caused by spasm of the cerebral arteries, the aura being due to cerebral ischaemia at this time, followed by vasodilatation which produces the headache. It may be precipitated by stress, certain foods or by the contraceptive pill.

Dyslexia

This is a disturbance in the ability to read. Although the child may be thought to have poor sight, appropriate testing will reveal normal visual acuities.

Hysterical Blindness

Occasionally, patients complain of poor sight but no abnormality can be found in the eyes or the central nervous system to account for their complaints. There may be a history of either family or personal problems. The patient may stand to gain from his 'blindness', e.g., financial compensation from the Criminal Injuries

Compensation Board or increased attention from his family. He may appear quite indifferent to his disability. The visual fields may become progressively smaller on testing ('spiral fields'). Such patients complaining of bilateral blindness still have normal pupil reactions and they tend not to fall over or bump into things.

Unilateral blindness may be disproved by eliciting a corrective movement when a prism is placed in front of the 'blind' eye. Other methods to catch the patient out depend upon confusing him with lenses so that he is not sure with which eye he is seeing.

Complete recovery is usual once the patient realises that his blindness has been disproved but he may later develop other hysterical manifestations.

21 SQUINT (STRABISMUS)

Introduction

A squint means that the visual axes of the two eyes do not meet on the object being observed. Normally, the eyes move as a pair, so that the maculae of both eyes are directed towards the object we wish to see. If this object is far away (6 metres or more) the visual axes of the two eyes are regarded as being parallel (i.e., they meet at infinity). If the object of interest is nearer, the visual axes meet at it. A squint means that the visual axis of one eye is not directed towards the object (Figure 21.1).

Figure 21.1: Squint

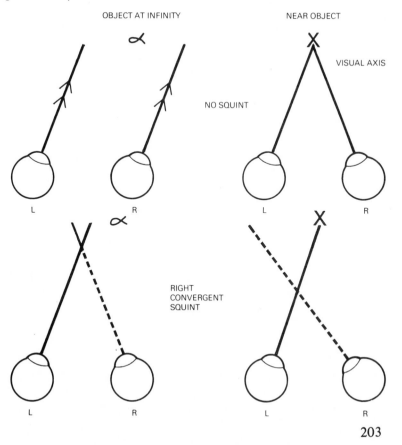

Binocular Single Vision

Normally the separate images formed on each retina are fused by the brain to produce a single mental 'picture'. This binocular single vision is an advantage, not only because it increases the field of vision and cancels out the blind spots of each eye but because it slightly improves the visual acuity and gives stereoscopic depth perception (i.e., '3-D' vision).

Binocular single vision is only possible provided each eye has a good visual acuity and the eyes are focused on the same object. In return, binocular single vision provides a 'reward' for keeping the eyes straight.

The Importance of Squint

A squint may be due to potentially lethal disorders, e.g., retinoblastoma (chapter 19), intracranial aneurysm (chapter 20). A squint means that binocular single vision is lost and diplopia may result. In small children the presence of a squint means that binocular single vision may never develop and one eye may become amblyopic. Effective treatment of these conditions is only possible if started during the early years of life. As soon as a squint is suspected the patient should be referred to an Eye Department.

The Causes of Squint

Central Causes

We learn to keep our eyes straight because this brings us the advantage of binocular single vision. A mentally retarded child may be unable to appreciate this advantage and therefore he often squints.

Paralytic Squint

A paralysed muscle makes it impossible for the eyes to move as a pair, so a squint results in certain directions of gaze (Figure 21.2). The palsy may be congenital or be due to trauma, dysthyroid eye disease, intracranial aneurysms (chapter 20) or diabetes.

Sensory Defects

If a retinoblastoma, cataract, corneal scar or a high refractive error in one eye prevents the formation of a clear retinal image, binocular vision can never be achieved, since the brain cannot fuse one clear and one blurred image.

Accommodative Squint

Accommodation and convergence (chapter 2) are linked together. The relationship is somewhat elastic but we cannot do one without the other, just as

Figure 21.2: Right Lateral Rectus Palsy

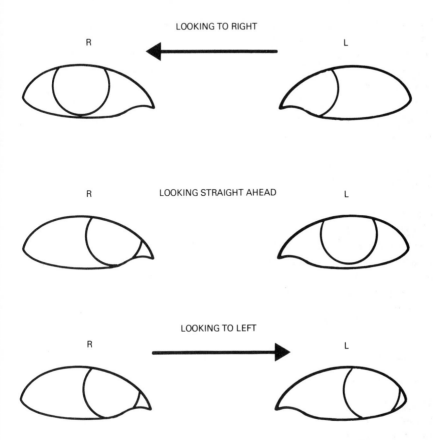

the little finger cannot be moved much without the ring finger being moved as well.

A child with hypermetropic eyes, who is exerting extra accommodation to see clearly, will inevitably be tending to converge his eyes. When he is well he may be able to control sufficiently his tendency to converge his eyes to obtain binocular single vision but an illness such as measles may cause him to lose control of the imbalance and a convergent squint may develop.

Types of Squint

A squint may be horizontal or vertical or both. Horizontal squints are either convergent (cross-eyed) or divergent (wall-eyed) (Figure 21.3).

Figure 21.3: Types of Squint

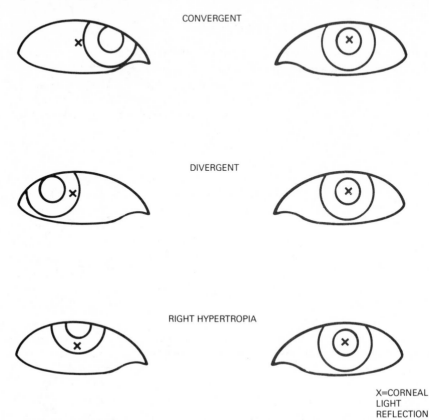

CONVERGENT

DIVERGENT

RIGHT HYPERTROPIA

X=CORNEAL
LIGHT
REFLECTION

In the case of vertical squints, one eye is directed above the other (e.g., left over right = L/R = left hypertropia; or right over left = R/L = right hypertropia). A squint may affect only one eye or alternate from one to the other (alternating squint). The angle of squint may be larger in one direction of gaze than in the opposite direction (incomitant or paralytic squint). The angle of squint may be the same in all directions of gaze (concomitant). The squint may be present all the time (manifest) or be present only some of the time (latent).

Consequences of a Squint

Diplopia

If the two eyes are not directed at the same object, differing retinal images will be presented to the brain and double vision will result. Diplopia is so distressing that patients find ways of avoiding it by shutting or patching one eye, adjusting the postion of their head appropriately or by suppressing the image seen with the squinting eye.

Compensatory Head Posture (CHP)

In the case of paralytic squints, the angle of squint varies with the direction of gaze, e.g., for a right lateral rectus palsy (Figure 21.2) there is no squint or diplopia when the patient looks to the left. By keeping his head turned to the right while viewing an object straight ahead, his eyes are turned leftwards and diplopia is avoided. However, a marked compensatory head posture looks odd and causes the patient discomfort.

Suppression and Amblyopia

All children with squints, and some adults too, are able to suppress the vision of one eye so that they do not see double. This suppression takes place in the brain. Whilst the visual pathways are still developing (this occurs during the first eight years or so of life) constant suppression of one eye will result in amblyopia (a 'lazy' eye). An amblyopic eye looks normal but it has a poor acuity (often 6/36 or less) which cannot be improved by glasses. An adult who suppresses the image of one eye retains good acuity in that eye. Children with alternating squints do not become amblyopic as each eye is used in turn.

Loss of Binocular Vision

A child who squints may never develop binocular single vision, or may permanently lose it, unless the squint is quickly corrected. An adult who squints loses binocular single vision all the time he is squinting.

Without binocular single vision, depth perception is much impaired although not completely absent. Some occupations become difficult and some are forbidden (e.g., flying an aeroplane). A child may be clumsier than he would otherwise be.

Cosmetic Considerations

Manifest squints, especially those of a large angle, are unsightly.

The Diagnosis of Squint

Some squints are obvious to everyone. Others are only diagnosed after several tests have been carried out and the patient has been seen on several occasions.

Popular Misconceptions about Squints

People may say that an individual squints because he screws up his eyes. It is important to find out exactly what the patient or his relatives notice wrong and explain what the term squint really means, if misunderstandings and unnecessary investigations are to be avoided. People often talk about 'growing out of a squint'. It is true that converging eyes tend to drift outwards with time so that a two-year-old child with a convergent squint may appear almost normal at ten years of age, but by this time he may have incurable amblyopia and have lost binocular single vision.

Figure 21.4: Epicanthus

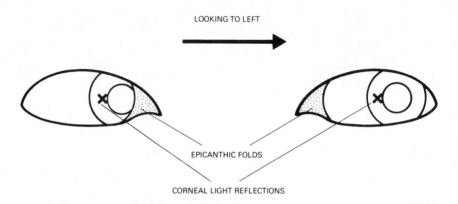

LOOKING TO LEFT

EPICANTHIC FOLDS

CORNEAL LIGHT REFLECTIONS

Children with epicanthus are often thought to have a squint, especially when they look sideways, but the eyes are in fact well aligned. The corneal light reflections are symmetrically placed (Figure 21.4). The appearance of the squint lessens as these children grow older because growth of the developing nose eliminates the skin folds, so ridding the child of the 'pseudo squint'. Of course, epicanthus and a true squint may co-exist.

Orthoptic Assessment

Visual Acuity (VA)

Even if the child cannot read a Snellen Chart, he may be able to match a letter on a card held by the Orthoptist 3 to 6 metres away from him with one of seven letters on a card which he himself holds (Sheridan Gardner Test).

Cover Tests (CT) (Figure 21.5)

These are used to demonstrate a squint which is not already obvious to the observer, to show up a latent squint, and to decide whether the squint is uniocular or alternating in nature.

Figure 21.5: Cover Test on Manifest Left Convergent Squint

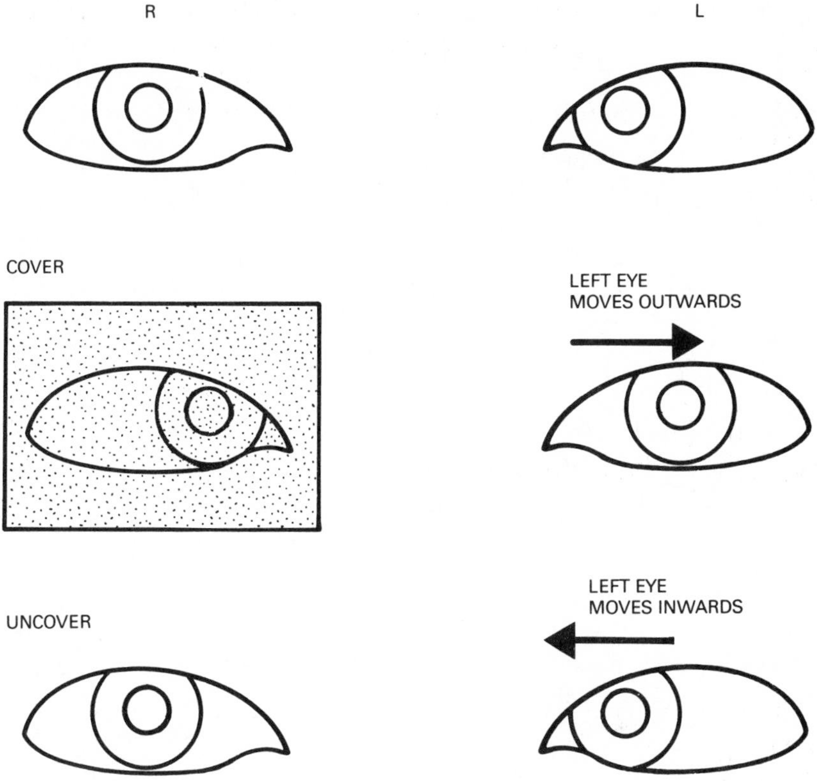

R

L

COVER

LEFT EYE
MOVES OUTWARDS

UNCOVER

LEFT EYE
MOVES INWARDS

External Ocular Movements (EOM)

Abnormalities of eye movements suggest that the squint is paralytic in origin.

Synoptophore (Major amblyoscope)

On this instrument the angle of squint is measured and the presence or absence of binocular single vision is determined.

Prism Cover Test (PCT)

This is another way of determining the angle of squint.

Wirt Fly

This is an alternative method of investigating binocular single vision.

Hess Chart

This piece of equipment is useful in studying patients with paralytic squint in order to determine which muscle is paralysed.

Management of Squint

Treatment of the Cause of Squint

It is only rarely that a squint is due to pathology such as a retinoblastoma, optic atrophy or a retinal detachment. Clearly in such instances, the underlying cause should receive appropriate treatment.

In the case of many children with squints, all that is necessary is the correction of refractive errors with glasses. Sometimes this step alone is sufficient to correct the squint and restore binocular single vision. Glasses may have to be worn indefinitely but sometimes they can be progressively weakened and finally completely discarded.

Treatment of Amblyopia

If the vision of one eye is not improved to a normal level by wearing the correct spectacles, the other eye is occluded (patched) to make the lazy one work. Initially, an opaque patch covering the whole eye is worn all day for a few weeks. Frequent orthoptic checks are made during this period as the covered eye occasionally becomes lazy itself (occlusion amblyopia). Once the acuity has been improved to a normal level, the occlusion may be reduced gradually until the patient is ready for surgery. When the vision of the two eyes is equal, the squint usually becomes alternating in character; unfortunately this may upset the parents who may complain that the squint has 'gone over to the other eye as well'.

Surgery

This may be carried out to achieve either a functional result (to restore binocular single vision in a child who has potential for it), or simply a cosmetic result — to make the child look better. Surgery for a functional result may be performed as soon as the patient is ready for it (once amblyopia has been corrected). If the surgeon is successful in straightening the eye the operation will probably be permanently successful because once binocular single vision is achieved, the child will want to keep it and will keep his eyes straight to retain it. Cosmetic surgery can be deferred for some time. The eyes are rarely straightened completely. Indeed, in the case of convergence squints, it is best to leave the eyes still slightly convergent. If they are quite straight, they may diverge over the years and the patient's plight may be worse, not better.

Operations are designed to strengthen muscles by resection, advancement, or tucking, or to weaken them by recession, myectomy, or tenotomy. For convergent squints, the lateral rectus muscles may be resected or the medial rectus muscles recessed. For divergent squints, the lateral rectus muscles are recessed and the medial rectus muscles resected. The amount of recession and resection depends upon the angle of squint and the surgeon's preference. Further surgery may be carried out once the effect of the first operation has become apparent.

Orthoptic Exercises

These help the patient to establish and maintain binocular single vision; they exercise voluntary convergence and they make the relationship between accommodation and convergence more flexible.

Prisms

Prisms bend rays of light. They do not correct a squint but they may be used to allow the two eyes to work together so that binocular single vision results (Figure 21.6). Glass prisms are thick and heavy so that only squints of a small angle can be treated with prisms incorporated in spectacles. Plastic stick-on Fresnel prisms can be used for squints of larger angles as they are thin and light but they blur vision so that they are useful only as a temporary expedient.

Special Points in the Treatment of Paralytic Squints

These squints tend to recover spontaneously so that it is usual to wait until there has been no change for six months before surgery is undertaken. Prisms are useful during the interim to restore binocular vision, but occasionally the only way to abolish diplopia is to patch one eye.

Illustrative Case History. John was three and a half years old. His parents first noticed a 'turn' in his right eye three months previously when he was recovering from measles. His General Practitioner referred him to a Consultant who confirmed the presence of a right convergent squint. The Orthoptist found visual acuities of right: 6/36; left: 6/6 (Sheridan Gardner test) and a right convergent squint measuring 25°. Cyclopentolate drops 1 per cent were instilled; the fundi were normal but an accurate refraction could not be carried out because he was so active. Consequently, a refraction was repeated at a further visit two weeks later after oc. atropine 1 per cent had been applied to both eyes at night time for the three days prior to the second visit. He was hypermetropic and lenses of +2.5 dioptre sphere were prescribed for each eye.

John was seen six weeks later in the Orthoptic Department. He had worn the glasses constantly since they had been collected from the Optician four weeks earlier but his vision was still VR: 6/36, VL: 6/6 and the squint measured 20°. The Orthoptist supplied elastoplast patches to be worn over the left eye all day. Four weeks later his vision was VR: 6/24, VL: 6/6 with spectacles and after a further six weeks, VR: 6/6 and VL: 6/6. The squint was now freely alternating and his name was entered on the waiting list for squint surgery. He continued to wear the glasses but patching was stopped.

On the day of admission he was seen by both the Orthoptist and the Surgeon; their findings were the same as at the last visit. The next day John was given a

Figure 21.6: a. Divergent Squint, b. 'Corrected' by a Prism

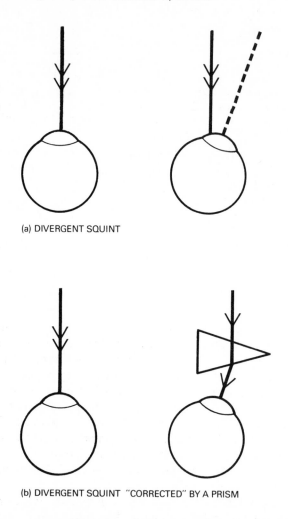

(a) DIVERGENT SQUINT

(b) DIVERGENT SQUINT "CORRECTED" BY A PRISM

general anaesthetic; his eyelids were cleaned and his head was draped in towels. Antibiotic drops were instilled in the right eye and a lid retractor inserted. Traction sutures were used to turn the eye laterally. The conjunctiva was incised over the medial rectus muscle and Tenon's capsule incised above and below the muscle insertion. A squint hook was placed beneath the muscle and the site of the tendon insertion was cleaned. Chromic catgut sutures were placed in the upper and lower borders of the tendon which was divided (Figure 21.7). The tendon was re-inserted 5mm back from its original insertion and the conjunctiva closed with plain collagen.

Figure 21.7: Medial Rectus Recession

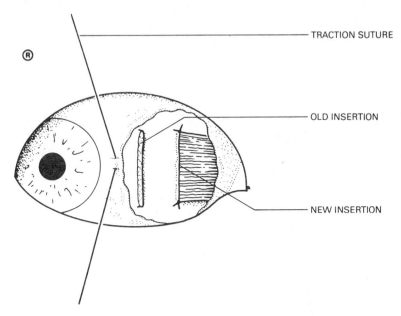

The eye was then turned medially by means of the traction sutures; the conjunctiva and Tenon's capsule were incised and the lateral rectus muscle was cleaned. Chromic cat gut sutures were placed in the muscle belly 5 mm back from the tendon insertion and 5 mm of the muscle was excised (Figure 21.8). The cut muscle was sutured to the original insertion and the conjunctiva was closed. An antibiotic ointment was applied. The eye was left unpadded.

Next day the eye was cleaned and antibiotic drops were instilled. He was seen by a doctor to check that there were no signs of infection and that the eye moved well in all directions. John was then allowed home. His parents were instructed to instil antibiotic drops three times daily for a week. They were told not to let John go swimming until he was next seen.

He was seen in the Orthoptic and Out-patient Departments a week after his discharge. The eye was healing well so the drops were stopped and the earlier restriction lifted.

At a follow-up appointment six weeks later, John's eyes were straight. He saw 6/6 with each eye, with and without glasses. The spectacles were discarded. At later appointments he was found to have binocular single vision. He was followed-up in the Orthoptic Department for some time. His eyes remained straight.

Figure 21.8: Lateral Rectus Resection

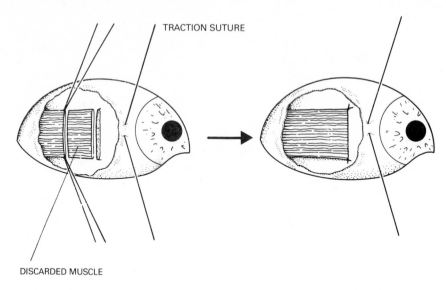

DISCARDED MUSCLE

Complications of Surgery

Infection. There is swelling of the eyelids and conjunctiva with purulent discharge and sometimes pyrexia. Local and systemic antibiotics are given and the child is kept in hospital until the infection begins to subside.

Stitch Granuloma. A red lump may persist over the muscle sutures and the parents may be concerned. However, the granuloma usually resolves over some weeks. Antibiotic or antibiotic and steroid drops may be prescribed. A persistent granuloma may need to be excised.

Conjunctival Separation. A minor gape may be ignored; otherwise resuturing of the conjunctiva under local or general anaesthesia is required.

Muscle Palsy. If a muscle suture comes untied, or cuts out of the sclera, there will be reduced movement of the eye in the immediate post-operative period. This must be corrected as soon as possible by re-attaching the muscle.

Under-or Over-correction. In the case of a convergent squint, under-correction results in persistence of the convergent squint and this may require a further operation — usually on the other eye. Over-correction results in consecutive divergence and requires re-operation to reverse the effect of the original operation. It should be noted that when the patient has no binocular vision, the eyes will never be exactly straight and the surgeon usually aims to slightly under-correct the malalignment of the eyes.

22 GENERAL DISORDERS AND THE EYE

Introduction

Many medical conditions affect the eye. Sometimes the patient's eyesight is threatened but often prompt treatment of the condition will preserve his vision. The changes in the eyes may be the first indication of the patient's illness. Some of the most common and important conditions are considered in this chapter.

Diabetes Mellitus

Diabetes affects about 2 per cent of the population of the United Kingdom and approximately 2 per cent of diabetics are blind because of their disease. Moreover, young people are often affected, rendering them unemployed and dependent upon others for their welfare.

Diabetic Retinopathy

Diabetes affects blood vessels throughout the body, including those in the retina. Two main types of retinopathy then develop — background retinopathy and proliferative retinopathy. Patients with retinopathy have usually been diabetic for many years.

Background Retinopathy ('Dot and Blot' Retinopathy). Microaneurysms (dots), haemorrhages (blots) and white exudates appear in the retina, where they are visible with the ophthalmoscope. Vision is not impaired unless the macula is affected by oedema due to leakage from normal vessels. Patients with such a maculopathy still retain peripheral vision and so may be relatively independent.

Proliferative Retinopathy. Although less common than background retinopathy, this is much more disabling. Both peripheral and central vision may be lost. New blood vessels develop in the retina (see p.173). A rete mirabile is a tuft of new vessels growing forwards from the optic disc. Vitreous haemorrhages ensue with temporary or permanent loss of vision (see p.170). Later fibrous tissue may grow out from the optic disc. Finally, the fibrous tissue contracts and a traction retinal detachment results.

Treatment of Retinopathy. Photocoagulation may be used to obliterate areas of hypoxic retina for it is currently thought that areas of retina that are poorly perfused with blood produce a chemical which leads to the sprouting of abnormal fronds of new vessels from the retinal circulation. This chemical, or vaso-proliferative factor, has not yet been isolated but the fact that ablation of hypoxic retina often leads to the regression of the tufts of neovascularisation certainly supports the proposed mechanism (chapter 19). If photocoagulation is used early enough, visual loss may be prevented. It is therefore essential that all diabetics have their fundi regularly examined under full mydriasis so that treatable retinopathy is detected at an early stage. Advanced cases are rarely helped by these means. Vitrectomy may be used to clear dense vitreous haemorrhages but the operation is particularly hazardous in diabetics and is obviously of no value if the retina is grossly diseased. Pituitary ablation by surgery or by irradiation is occasionally used in severe retinopathy. Clofibrate tablets clear exudates but do not improve vision. Good control of the diabetes is desirable but retinopathy may progress despite it.

Cataract

Senile cataracts are common in diabetics but probably not much more common than in the general population. Cataract extraction in diabetics carries more hazards both to the eye and to the patient's general health. It is also less likely to give good visual results because diabetics so often have a co-existing retinopathy. True diabetic cataract is rare. It is usually seen at the onset of the disease when the blood sugar level is high. Sugars enter the lens and water follows by osmotic attraction. The lens fibres swell and burst and the lens rapidly becomes opaque. Cataract extraction is then required and in young people is usually performed by the extracapsular technique.

Refractive Errors

These develop when the blood sugar level is unstable. Hyperglycaemia, causes swelling of the lens; this makes the patient myopic. Further lens swelling leads to cataract formation (see above). Hypoglycaemia, due to energetic treatment, causes hypermetropia.

A patient requiring frequent changes of glasses should, therefore, be investigated for diabetes. Similarly, glasses should not be prescribed for a recently diagnosed diabetic until the condition is well controlled.

Rubeosis

This is a condition in which abnormal new blood vessels develop on the iris and in the drainage angle. It occurs most commonly in association with diabetes and central retinal vein occlusion and is due to hypoxia within the eye. It is usually followed by an intractable form of glaucoma which may necessitate enucleation (see p.144).

Nerve Palsy

Loss of function of the third or sixth cranial nerves with resultant squint and diplopia may be due to diabetes affecting the nutrient vessels supplying the nerves (see p.204).

Practical Considerations

Diabetics in Out-patients. Diabetics who have been waiting a long time in the Department may need a snack or meal to prevent a hypoglycaemic attack. Most diabetics will need to have their pupils dilated at some stage so that retinopathy may be sought. Similarly, fluorescein angiography is often performed to delineate new vessels or areas of ischaemic retina. Many diabetics are first diagnosed in Ophthalmic Out-patient Departments when patients with refractive changes, cataracts or retinal vascular disease have their urine tested.

Diabetics on the Ward. On admission, details of insulin and other treatment and normal meal times should be ascertained. As far as possible these should be maintained in hospital. The patient's urine must be tested regularly. Any operation is normally postponed if there is ketonuria or over 2 per cent glycosuria. Areas of sepsis on the feet must be sought and treated. Diabetics with poor sight may be unable to read their insulin syringes and so require supervision.

Operations on Diabetics. The anaesthetist determines what treatment is necessary on the day of operation. Usually the insulin dosage is halved and drugs, such as chlorpropamide, omitted. Diabetics should be first on the operating list. Blood glucose is usually checked on the day of operation and post-operatively as required. Anaesthesia masks the signs of hypoglycaemia, so that it is vital that the blood glucose does not fall too low during the operation. A dextrose infusion may be given if the operation is prolonged. It is usually possible for the patient to resume his normal diet soon after the operation so that his routine need not be greatly disturbed. He is discharged home as soon as his diabetes is stable and his eye condition satisfactory.

Complications of Operation. Bleeding of the tissues often makes an operation on a diabetic eye more difficult. Hyphaema, vitreous haemorrhage and retinal haemorrhages may occur post-operatively; extra rest is usually advised. Chest infection, urinary tract infection and bed sores may also prolong the patient's stay in hospital.

Hypertension

Hypertension affects the eyes because the retinal blood vessels become diseased. Occasionally, hypertension is first diagnosed on examination of the fundi and confirmed with the sphygmomanometer. The appearance of the fundi gives some guide to the severity of the hypertension. In mild cases, the arteries may appear thinner and shinier with the ophthalmoscope. The veins may appear constricted where they are crossed by the arteries (arterio-venous or 'A-V' nipping). In severe hypertension flame-shaped haemorrhages and micro-infarcts ('cotton wool spots') may appear in the retina. In malignant hypertension (which is fatal if left untreated), papilloedema also develops and the patient may experience blurring of vision. These signs and symptoms may resolve completely if the hypertension is treated promptly.

Pre-eclampsia (Toxaemia of Pregnancy)

Hypertensive retinopathy with blurring of vision may develop in this condition. In severe cases serous detachment of the retina may complicate the retinopathy (see p.185). It is usually necessary to expedite delivery if these ocular changes develop.

Thyroid Disease and the Eye

The thyroid gland controls the basal metabolic rate by secreting the hormone thyroxine.

A deficiency of thyroxine (hypothyroidism) may be associated with thickening of the skin (myxoedema) including that of the eyelids.

An excess of thyroxine (thyrotoxicosis or Graves's disease) may be associated with characteristic and potentially serious changes of the eyes. Indeed, thyrotoxicosis may be first diagnosed in the Ophthalmic Out-patient Department. However, most of these eye changes are due, not to an excess of thyroxine, but to an abnormality of other hormones. Thus, identical changes sometimes occur when the thyroxine levels are actually normal or reduced. The condition may then be termed ophthalmic Graves's disease or dysthyroid eye disease.

Dysthyroid Eye Disease

The most striking feature of this condition is protrusion of one or both eyes (exophthalmos). The staring appearance that this creates is increased by retraction of the eyelids, a tendency for the lids to lag behind the globe on down gaze and infrequent blinking. All these features may lead to exposure keratitis with disastrous effects on the patient's vision (see p.116). Exophthalmos is due to swelling of the orbital tissues, including the extraocular muscles. The enlarged muscles become inefficient so that defective eye movement and diplopia may develop. Finally the swollen muscles may compress the optic nerve, causing reduced vision and eventually optic atrophy.

Treatment

These eye changes may be unaffected or even be worsened by treatment of the thyrotoxicosis, especially if the patient becomes hypothyroid as a result of treatment. The best that can be done is to achieve a normal, euthyroid, state. Systemic steroids, given with antithyroid drugs, may reduce the exophthalmos.

Lateral tarsorrhaphies may be necessary to prevent or to treat exposure keratitis; they may also improve the cosmetic appearance. When damage to the optic nerve is threatened, surgical decompression of the orbit should be considered. This is probably best achieved by removing either the lateral or medial wall of the orbit so that the orbital tissues can expand, so relieving the pressure on the optic nerve.

Giant Cell Arteritis (Temporal Arteritis)

In this disease arteries become inflamed and, ultimately, become occluded. As a result the patient may suffer infarction of the heart, brain or gut. The temporal arteries are commonly affected causing them to become tender and thickened. The patient may then complain of pain on chewing, or brushing his hair. The eyes are often affected; vision is lost suddenly and permanently in one eye due to occlusion of the posterior ciliary arteries; this results in an ischaemic optic neuropathy (see p.187). Occasionally, a central retinal artery occlusion is the cause of visual loss. There may have been warning transient ischaemic attacks beforehand. Without treatment loss of vision of the other eye is likely to follow. Occasionally, nerve palsies with associated diplopia occur.

Investigations

An Erythrocyte Sedimentation Rate (ESR) should be performed immediately the disease is suspected; typically the reading is markedly raised. A biopsy of a temporal artery may then be performed under local anaesthesia. If it shows typical inflammation with giant cells, the diagnosis is confirmed. However, treatment must be started immediately, before the result of the biopsy is available.

Treatment

Systemic steroids are given in large doses until the ESR is normal. They must be continued for as long as the disease is active. The dose is judged on the patient's symptoms and on the ESR, which is performed at regular intervals. The penalty for discontinuing treatment prematurely is sudden blindness in the other eye.

Sarcoidosis

This disease is most commonly seen in young women; often they are Negroes from the West Indies. The cause is unknown. It may affect many structures including the lungs, skin and kidneys. Severe chronic cases may develop renal failure, pulmonary fibrosis and heart failure.

Ocular Changes

About 15 per cent of patients with sarcoidosis have ocular changes. Iritis, either acute or chronic, is common. Typically, it is granulomatous with 'mutton fat' keratic precipitates, iris nodules and broad posterior synechiae (see p.125). Choroiditis, swelling of the optic discs, and retinal vasculitis (see p.174) also occur. The eyes are commonly dry. Rarely the lacrimal glands are grossly enlarged due to chronic dacryoadenitis (chapter 11).

Investigations

Sarcoidosis is sometimes first diagnosed during the investigation of a patient with iritis. Features suggestive of sarcoidosis are hilar lymphadenopathy on chest X-ray, a negative Mantoux test and elevated serum or urinary calcium levels. The diagnosis may be confirmed by a Kveim Test; this entails the injection of Kveim antigen into the forearm and biopsy of the injected skin six weeks later. A typical microscopic reaction should develop.

Treatment

There is no cure for sarcoidosis; however, it may improve spontaneously. Systemic steroids may be needed for severe iritis or pulmonary fibrosis. Milder forms of iritis are treated in the usual way with steroid and mydriatic drops. Dry eyes are treated with artificial tears.

Tuberculosis

Now that tuberculosis has become uncommon in the United Kingdom its ophthalmic manifestations are rarely seen in this country. However, they include nodules in the conjunctiva, iris or choroid and optic atrophy and iritis. A patient with any of these changes should have his chest X-rayed because tuberculosis is infectious and can be fatal. It may be worsened if systemic steroids are given as part of his ophthalmic treatment.

Some anti-tuberculous drugs (e.g., ethambutol) may cause optic atrophy.

Syphilis

Syphilis is also uncommon nowadays but its ophthalmic manifestations may still be seen because they are often long lasting. Secondary syphilis (which develops a few months after infection) may cause iritis. Since syphilis may be cured by antibiotic treatment at this stage, appropriate blood tests (e.g., VDRL) should be performed on every patient with iritis. Tertiary syphilis, which develops years after infection, may be associated with optic atrophy and Argyll-

Robertson pupils (see p.197). Congenital syphilis may lead to interstitial keratitis. The initial phase of acute keratitis is a painful condition. It is followed by corneal scarring, which may necessitate grafting (see p.115).

Myasthenia Gravis

This disease causes weakness of the voluntary muscles. The basic abnormality lies at the junctions between the motor nerves and the muscles they innervate (the neuro-muscular junctions). Anticholinesterase drugs are usually beneficial. They increase the amount of acetylcholine present at the neuro-muscular junctions by inhibiting the enzyme cholinesterase (chapter 2). Thus it may be that insufficient acetylcholine is released by the motor nerves or that its uptake by the muscles is impaired.

Signs and Symptoms

The weakness may affect the skeletal muscles causing weakness of the limbs, the pharyngeal muscles causing difficulty in swallowing, or the muscles of the eye causing ptosis, squint and diplopia. The disease is occasionally fatal because of involvement of the respiratory muscles. Characteristically, myasthenic muscles become weaker as the day goes on but recover with rest.

Diagnosis

The Tensilon test is performed by exercising a weak muscle (e.g., the levator palpebrae) until it becomes fatigued and then injecting the anticholinesterase drug edrophonium (Tensilon) intravenously. If the weakness is due to myasthenia the ptosis will be rapidly (but temporarily) abolished. This test can be dangerous so that facilities for resuscitating the patient should be available.

Treatment

Anticholinesterase drugs (neostigmine, pyridostigmine) are given by mouth. Thymectomy may produce an improvement if performed early in the course of the disease. Ptosis may be helped by props on contact lenses or spectacle frames. Surgery for ptosis or squint should be avoided if possible since general anaesthesia may precipitate a worsening of the disease.

23 TRAUMA

Traumatic cases form a large part of the work-load of the Ophthalmic Casualty Department. It is imperative that the visual acuity of both eyes of the patient be measured at the first and last attendances as this will provide important information in any legal proceedings that may ensue.

Blunt Trauma

The eye and its appendages may be seriously damaged by a variety of blunt objects, such as fists, elbows, squash balls, etc. Those that fit within the orbital rim and which travel very fast (e.g., squash balls and champagne corks) cause the greatest damage. The eye should be carefully examined from front to back for the following injuries, remembering that one lesion may hide another.

Periorbital Haematoma (Black Eye)

Swelling and bruising of the lids may be severe and progressive. It subsides spontaneously in a few days but the eye must be inspected for underlying damage before discharging the patient from the Casualty Department.

Subconjunctival Haemorrhage (Figure 23.1)

These haemorrhages of themselves are harmless and require no treatment but if the posterior edge of the haemorrhage cannot be seen (Figure 23.2), a skull fracture should be suspected and the patient be X-rayed. They may also obscure a scleral perforation.

Figure 23.1: Subconjunctival Haemorrhage

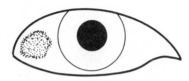

Corneal Abrasion (Figure 23.3)

This may be caused by a baby's finger nail, by the patient vigorously rubbing his eye in an attempt to remove a foreign body, or by excessive contact lens wear. The eye is very painful and the patient may not allow anyone to examine it until

222

Figure 23.2: Subconjunctival Haemorrhage Complicating Skull Fracture

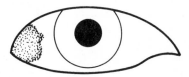

local anaesthetic drops have been instilled to relieve him of his agony. The abraded area of the corneal epithelium stains bright green with fluorescein.

Antibiotic drops should be instilled or ointment applied and the eye padded and bandaged for 24 hours. The eye is inspected daily to check for infection and the dressing repeated until the cornea has healed. Analgesic tablets may be required. A short-acting mydriatic (e.g., guttae homatropine 1 to 2 per cent) may also be used to relieve pain from the ciliary spasm which accompanies large abrasions.

Figure 23.3: Corneal Abrasion

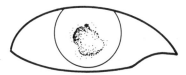

Hyphaema

This is the term given to blood in the anterior chamber (Figure 23.4). The bleeding arises from torn vessels in the iris or on the anterior surface of the ciliary body.

Figure 23.4: Hyphaema

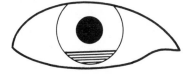

Management. The patient should be admitted for bed rest. Steroid drops are instilled to minimise the tendency to intraocular inflammation. No miotics or mydriatics are given until the blood has absorbed. Then the pupil is dilated and the fundus examined. The patient may be discharged after four or five days but should be seen in the clinic on a long-term basis as there is a risk of chronic glaucoma developing in the injured eye. This is particularly true if the angle structures have been torn (angle recession).

Complications. There is a considerable risk of re-bleeding occurring three days after the injury. This secondary bleed may be larger than the first; a total hyphaema is not uncommon. Bleeding may be so profuse that the intraocular pressure rises. The arterial blood supply to the eye may be reduced because of this pressure, so that the oxygen level in the eye falls and the total hyphaema becomes black — 'black ball hyphaema'. Some patients do not present until this occurs.

A black ball hyphaema causes severe pain. If the pressure remains high, it may force blood into the cornea, causing staining which obscures vision, and which may not clear for years. Acetazolamide is given to lower the intraocular pressure and oral analgesics are required. If the pressure remains very high an anterior chamber wash-out may be advised. This may, however, be accompanied by further bleeding and other operative complications.

Iris Injuries (Figure 23.5)

These are frequently accompanied by a hyphaema. Mydriasis may be temporary or permanent. It may cause annoying photophobia. The periphery of the iris is particularly thin and it is readily torn. Should this happen in one quadrant (iridodialysis) then the pupil becomes 'D' shaped.

Figure 23.5 Iris Injuries

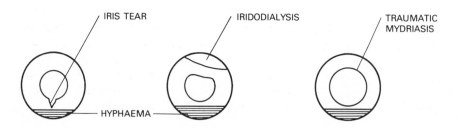

Angle Recession

This is a partial split in the drainage angle which causes it to become wider. It is frequently found in patients who have had a hyphaema. It is detected on gonioscopy. Chronic glaucoma may develop later because of the angle damage.

Lens Injuries

The lens may subluxate, dislocate or develop opacities (chapter 17). A rosette cataract is characteristic of blunt trauma (Figure 23.6).

Figure 23.6: Rosette Cataract

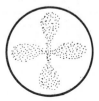

Ciliary Body Injury

Severe damage to the ciliary body may cause failure of aqueous production and hypotony. Thus, a severely damaged eye may eventually become phthisical.

Vitreous Haemorrhage

This may arise from bleeding from the ciliary body or the retina. It takes much longer to clear than a hyphaema (which may obscure it initially) and carries a worse prognosis for vision.

Retinal Damage (Figure 23.7)

Milky white patches in the central or peripheral retina are due to oedema and are given the name 'commotio retinae'. The oedema clears spontaneously but may be followed by the development of a retinal tear or permanent scarring in the affected area. Tears frequently lead to the development of a retinal detachment. Macular scarring causes a permanent reduction of the visual acuity. Retinal haemorrhages and tears may be seen immediately after the injury.

Choroidal Damage

Tears in the choroid and overlying retina tend to form part of a circle around the disc and may cause profound loss of vision if the papillo-macular bundle is damaged (Figure 23.8).

Figure 23.7: Retinal Injuries

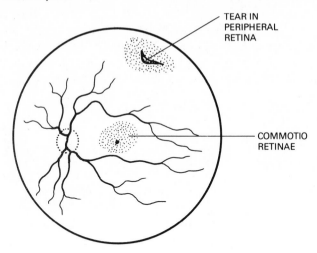

Figure 23.8: Choroidal Rupture

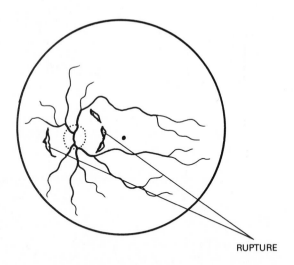

Optic Nerve Damage

The optic nerve may be torn from the eye causing instant blindness. An injury to the vascular supply of the nerve may be responsible for an unresponsive pupil and the development of a pale optic disc and blindness a few weeks later.

Blow-out Fracture of the Orbit

A sudden rise in the pressure within the orbit from a blow may cause a fracture of one of the egg-shell thin orbital walls. It is usually the floor of the orbit that gives way. Initially, bruising and swelling of the lids may mask the signs of a blow-out fracture. As the bruising subsides, enophthalmos and restricted eye movements with diplopia become apparent. The latter are due to entrapment of muscles or their fascia in the fracture. X-rays show an opaque maxillary antrum and sometimes a 'hanging drop' sign (Figure 23.9). This is due to orbital contents hanging down through the roof of the antrum.

A severe blow-out fracture may necessitate an operation to correct the enophthalmos for cosmetic reasons. Less severe cases may require squint surgery to correct diplopia. Many cases resolve sufficiently for surgery not to be warranted.

Figure 23.9: Blow-out Fracture of the Orbit; Hanging Drop Sign

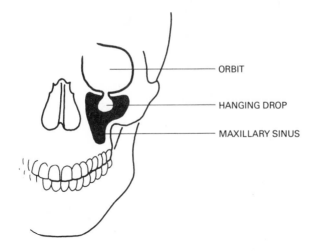

Penetrating Trauma

Road traffic accidents, warfare or the careless use of scissors, knives or darts (especially by children) are responsible for most of these injuries. If the patient has other major injuries the serious nature of his eye injury may be overlooked at first. However, early repair is essential and should take priority over treatment of other wounds and fractures unless they are life threatening.

Lid Lacerations

These may appear quite trivial and yet may be full-thickness wounds with underlying damage to the eye, orbit or even the brain. Injuries to the medial part of the lid may be associated with trauma to the canaliculi with the risk of permanent epiphora. Upper lid lacerations may involve the levator muscle with the risk of permanent ptosis. Injuries to the lid margin may be followed by trichiasis, entropion or ectropion if they are badly repaired.

The lid wounds must be thoroughly explored under general anaesthesia, if necessary, and meticulously repaired by an eye surgeon. A silicone tube (O'Donaghue's) may be inserted as an internal splint for a torn lower canaliculus and retained until healing has occurred (Figure 23.10). Intubation is sometimes achieved by threading a pigtail probe through the canaliculi, tying the silicone tube to it and then pulling the tube through the canaliculi as the probe is withdrawn. Torn upper canaliculi are less likely to result in epiphora. As passing a pigtail probe can damage the all-important lower canaliculus where the upper canaliculus alone is torn, the upper lid is usually repaired without intubation. Some surgeons do not attempt intubation, relying upon exact apposition of the cut ends of the canaliculus, which can be achieved under the operating microscope, to lead to patency of the tear passage.

Figure 23.10: Repair of Torn Canaliculis

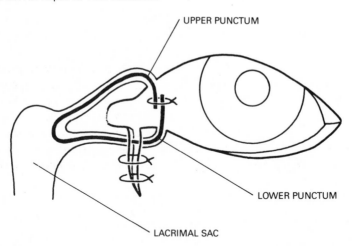

UPPER PUNCTUM

LOWER PUNCTUM

LACRIMAL SAC

Conjunctival Lacerations

These again may appear trivial and yet hide a scleral laceration. They should be explored under local or general anaesthesia and be sutured.

Lacerations of the Globe

These may be corneal or scleral, full thickness (perforating) or partial thickness. Minor corneal perforations may seal themselves spontaneously. Larger perforations are usually associated with prolapse of the iris. Hyphaema and lens damage are frequent accompaniments (Figure 23.11). Scleral perforations are often associated with prolapse of uveal tissue or vitreous. Combined corneo-scleral perforations carry the worst prognosis; the lens, vitreous and part of the uveal tract may all be involved.

Figure 23.11: Iris Prolapse

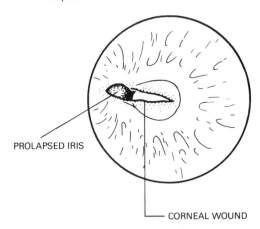

PROLAPSED IRIS

CORNEAL WOUND

Management

It is usually advisable to X-ray the orbit to exclude any intraocular foreign bodies. As soon as the patient is fit for an anaesthetic he is taken to the operating theatre and the eye is cleaned and explored. Prolapsed uvea and vitreous are abscised; lens matter and blood are washed away and the corneal and scleral lacerations are carefully sutured. The anterior chamber is reformed with air or saline and an antibiotic is injected beneath the conjunctiva. Any lacrimal, lid or facial lacerations may then be repaired. Tetanus toxoid and systemic antibiotics may be required.

Complications

Infection (see chapter 17)

Cataract. This may develop very rapidly and cause the lens to swell. Early re-operation to wash out the lens matter may be necessary.

Retinal Detachment. This frequently occurs after a scleral perforation which was complicated by damage to the retina or by bleeding into the vitreous.

Corneal Scarring and Irregularity. Meticulous repair of the cornea with fine nylon sutures should achieve a watertight wound. The surgeon also aims to keep subsequent scarring to a minimum and to so place the sutures that the normal corneal curvature is restored; otherwise marked astigmatism may result which will lead to a poor visual acuity.

Sympathetic Ophthalmia (chapter 15). This is the rarest but the most feared complication. It is a bilateral, chronic uveitis that follows a perforating injury of one eye. The inflammation starts in the injured eye and involves the second eye about eight weeks after the injury. However, this time span is variable. Intervals of five days to fifty years have been recorded. Although steroids will reduce the inflammation, the patient may eventually become completely blind in both eyes. For this reason, most surgeons prefer to enucleate any injured eye which retains little useful vision, especially if the eye is persistently inflamed. Enucleation should be carried out within ten days of the injury. Once sympathetic ophthalmia has developed in the fellow eye, enucleation of the injured eye does not affect the course of the inflammation in the remaining eye.

Penetrating Wounds of the Orbit

The orbital walls are thin and may be easily breached by a knife, stick or bullet. Damage to the underlying meninges, brain or intracranial vessels may have fatal consequences through meningitis or intracranial bleeding.

Foreign Bodies

These may drop into the eye (e.g., from a ceiling or from beneath a car), blow in (on a windy day), or enter with considerable force whilst the patient is using an industrial grinding machine or a hammer and chisel. It is important to take a good history and an X-ray examination is mandatory in order to identify or exclude intraocular foreign bodies in all those instances in which the presence of a retained foreign body is a possibility.

Subtarsal and corneal foreign bodies are often far more painful than an intraocular foreign body. Discomfort and foreign body sensation due to conjunctival and corneal abrasions may persist after the foreign body has been dislodged by lacrimation or by rubbing the eye.

Conjunctival Foreign Body

Most foreign bodies striking the conjunctiva are quickly washed away by the tears, but molten metal may adhere to the ocular tissues and it may be necessary to pick the metal off with forceps.

Subtarsal Foreign Body

A foreign body may lodge beneath the upper tarsal plate. This may be removed with a cotton bud after eversion of the upper lid (chapter 5). An antibiotic ointment should be applied and the patient discharged.

Corneal Foreign Bodies

These cause pain, watering and photophobia. Such foreign bodies are commonly metallic and are rust coloured. Fluorescein drops tend to pool around a foreign body rendering it more clearly visible. If not removed immediately, the foreign body causes a white ring of corneal oedema to develop and this helps to loosen the fragment. Local anaesthetic drops should be instilled and the foreign body removed with a sharp needle using a slit-lamp microscope or magnifying glasses. If the deepest portion of the associated 'rust ring' remains tightly adherent it is better to leave it to loosen spontaneously rather than to risk causing further corneal damage by attempting to remove it. An antibiotic ointment and a pad and bandage are applied. The eye is examined daily and further removal of the 'rust ring' is attempted if necessary. The dressings are repeated until the eye has healed. A small scar is inevitable after removal of a deeply embedded foreign body but this affects vision only if it is at the centre of the cornea.

Intraocular Foreign Body

Any symptoms and signs may be minimal unless the foreign body is relatively large. However, the patient gives a history of something entering the eye with considerable force. Careful examination may reveal a corneal wound, iris perforation, early cataract formation or the foreign body itself lodged in the drainage angle, the lens, vitreous or on the retina.

Consequences. Non-metallic foreign bodies (e.g., wood) commonly cause infection within the eye, often with disastrous consequences. Metallic foreign bodies are frequently sterile but if they contain iron or copper a chemical reaction is set up which may be just as damaging as an infection. Intraocular iron poisons the neuroretina causing progressive blindness. In addition, the iris may become brown and a cataract develop — a condition known as siderosis. Intraocular copper may result in an acute sterile endophthalmitis developing or in a progressive greenish staining of intraocular membranes and the lens with cataract formation (chalcosis).

Management. Special X-ray techniques are used to localise the intraocular foreign body within the eye. Usually, a metal limbal ring (incorporated in a contact lens) is applied to the eye and X-rays repeated so that the position of the foreign body can be deduced (Figure 23.12). Removal of the foreign body is attempted under general anaesthesia. An appropriate corneal or scleral incision is made and the foreign body extracted with a giant magnet or with intraocular forceps (if the foreign body is non-magnetic). The wound is repaired and treatment continued as for a perforating eye injury. A foreign body retained in the lens itself should be dealt with by lens extraction.

Prognosis. This is often poor, despite the successful removal of the foreign body, for cataract formation and retinal detachment are common sequelae.

Figure 23.12: Intraocular Foreign Body Location

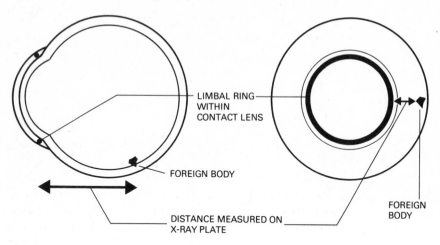

LIMBAL RING
WITHIN
CONTACT LENS

FOREIGN BODY

DISTANCE MEASURED ON
X-RAY PLATE

FOREIGN
BODY

Chemical Injuries

Patients attend Casualty with injuries due to a wide variety of chemicals entering their eyes. Strong alkalis, such as caustic soda (contained in oven cleaners), cause the most profound damage as they rapidly penetrate the cornea and damage the intraocular tissues. First-aid treatment for chemical burns consists of prompt and copious irrigation of the eye with water. Irrigation should be repeated in the Casualty Department using universal buffer solution or normal saline.

The extent of the damage is then assessed, after the instillation of a drop of local anaesthetic if necessary. Any solid particles of chemicals should be removed with forceps. Large corneal and conjunctival abrasions are often found. It may be necessary to admit the patient to hospital and to continue treatment with prolonged irrigation of the eye from an intravenous giving set. Further treatment with local steroids, antibiotic ointment and mydriatics is routine. Daily 'rodding' of the conjunctival fornices or insertion of a moulded scleral contact lens may be required to try and prevent the development of conjunctival adhesions.

Complications of Chemical Burns

These include conjunctival and corneal scarring with dryness of the eyes and deformities of the lids. Prolonged follow up and treatment of these complications may still fail to prevent blindness, and corneal grafts are often unsuccessful in these cases, usually because the cornea becomes vascularised as a result of the injury.

Thermal Injuries

Burns of the lids are potentially very serious because of the risk of corneal exposure. The cornea may be adequately covered at first but become exposed later because burnt tissue contracts as it heals. Emergency skin grafting may be necessary.

Ultra-violet Light Injury

Prolonged sunbathing, exposure to ultra-violet lamps without protective goggles and 'arc eye' (welder's flash) cause a similar pattern of corneal damage. Typically the patient is symptom-free at first but several hours after exposure to the damaging radiation, he complains of severe pain in one or both eyes. Fluorescein staining of the cornea shows multiple tiny defects — superficial punctate keratopathy (SPK) (Figure 23.13). Oral analgesics are prescribed to control the pain. Local treatment is as for a corneal abrasion. The epithelium usually heals in 24 to 48 hours.

Figure 23.13: Superficial Punctate Keratopathy

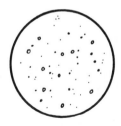

Infra-red Light Injury

'Solar maculopathy' follows prolonged gazing at the sun or viewing an eclipse of the sun without adequate protection of the eye. Treatment is of no avail. The visual acuity may be markedly and permanently impaired.

24 REMOVAL OF THE EYE

Indications

1. To save life (e.g., in the case of retinoblastoma).
2. To save sight in the other eye — prevention of sympathetic ophthalmia (chapter 15).
3. To relieve pain and to improve the appearance (e.g., in thrombotic glaucoma, phthisi bulbi, or a severely injured blind eye).

Staff Opinions

When an eye with some sight is to be removed at least two Consultants should record in the notes their opinion that this is necessary.

Enucleation

This is removal of the eyeball and its contents. This procedure is contra-indicated in the case of panophthalmitis because infection may spread to the meninges and subarachnoid space when the optic nerve is cut. Enucleation is usually carried out under general anaesthesia.

Method

Antibiotic drops are instilled into the conjunctival sac and a lid retractor is inserted. The conjunctiva is incised around the limbus and dissected off the globe. The rectus muscles are isolated and divided after a suture has been placed in each muscle. The globe is drawn forwards with forceps and the optic nerve clamped briefly before being cut. (This lessens bleeding.) The globe is removed and sent for histological examination and the socket packed with hot swabs to arrest any bleeding. The muscles are sutured together, preferably over an implant (Figure 24.1). Tenon's capsule and the conjunctiva are closed in layers. An antibiotic ointment is applied and the lids closed, ensuring that the lashes are not turned inwards. A pressure pad is secured with a bandage around the head.

Removal of Donor Eyes for Corneal Grafting (chapter 13)

Enucleation is carried out as above but there is no need to suture the muscles or conjunctiva or to clamp the optic nerve. Artificial eyes may be inserted or the lids

234

Figure 24.1: Implant

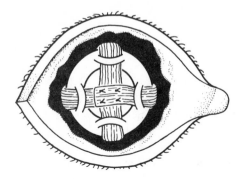

sutured together with hidden buried sutures so that the body does not appear mutilated.

Evisceration

This is removal of the contents of the globe, leaving the sclera and optic nerve behind. It is mainly used for treating cases of panophthalmitis. It is contra-indicated in the case of intraocular tumours and for the prevention of sympathetic ophthalmia because particles of uveal tissue may be left attached to the sclera.

Method

The conjunctiva is incised at the limbus. The cornea and a rim of sclera are excised and the contents of the globe scraped out very thoroughly with a Mules evisceration scoop. The scleral shell is filled with ointment. Tenon's capsule and the conjunctiva may be closed in layers or left open.

Aftercare

The first dressing is done at 48 hours. The lids are cleaned and drops are instilled into the socket. If there is no bleeding, dark glasses may be provided and the patient discharged. A transparent shell is fitted a few days later (Figure 24.2). This keeps the lids everted, preventing irritation of the socket by the lashes and accustoms the patient to having something in the socket. The antibiotic drops are continued.

The patient should visit the Artificial Eye Fitter about four weeks later. The fitter supplies a temporary artificial eye which nearly matches the patient's remaining eye for colour of the sclera and iris and also pupil size. He orders a permanent eye, individually painted according to a detailed description. This may be either a shell or a moulded eye. The latter requires an impression of the socket

Figure 24.2: Shell

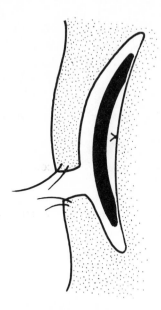

to be taken and a mould prepared.

Modern artificial eyes are made of acrylic and they are relatively non-irritant but they always cause a small amount of discharge from the socket. This should be wiped away each morning. It is not necessary to remove an artificial eye except for medical examination. Removal is easily accomplished using a plastic lever which is inserted under the lower edge of the prosthesis. Once this edge is dislodged over the lower lid the artificial eye slips out. For re-insertion, the artificial eye is positioned with the most pointed end towards the nose and the more rounded upper edge inserted under the upper lid (Figure 24.3). Artificial eyes need repolishing or replacing at intervals, so that patients should have regular appointments with the fitter.

Good movement of an artificial eye is best achieved when an implant has been used. The incorporation of magnets in both the implant and the artificial eye may result in an enhanced range of movement. Discomfort in a socket may be due to extrusion of an implant. Occasionally an artificial eye keeps falling out. This may be due to lid laxity or shrinkage of the socket. The former may warrant a lateral tarsorrhaphy; the latter may require conjunctival grafting.

Exenteration

This is removal of the contents of the bony orbit — the globe, muscles, lids and lacrimal gland. It is a mutilating operation used for intraocular tumours which

Figure 24.3: Left Artificial Eye

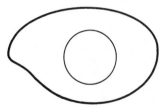

have spread outside the globe or for advanced lid and lacrimal gland tumours.

After the operation the defect may be covered with a pad, black patch or a prosthesis attached to a spectacle frame. Unless the orbit has been lined with a skin graft, regular cleaning of the resultant cavity is required.

25 BLIND REGISTRATION AND CARE OF THE BLIND

Blind Registration

The Consultant Ophthalmologist may register a patient as blind if the corrected visual acuity is less than 3/60 in the better eye or less than 6/36 if there is extensive associated visual field loss. Many patients are reluctant to be registered, although such registration does not imply that they are, or will become, totally blind. Registration of partial sight is carried out in the same way if the patient's corrected visual acuity is less than 6/36 in the better eye or 6/18 with marked reduction in the visual fields.

The Consultant fills in a Form BD.8 which is posted to the Social Services Department. An area social worker visits the patient, assesses his needs and delivers a large-print book setting out the services available to the visually handicapped. The following help may be offered.

Financial Benefits (Only for Those Registered Blind)

These include higher supplementary benefit, higher rent and rate allowances, higher tax allowance, reduced television licence fee, free radio loan, concessionary rates for travel on British Rail for the blind person and his companion, orange disablement parking disc and free post-aural hearing aids (if required).

Retraining For Employment

The young blind may be sent on special courses at Torquay by the blind person's resettlement officer, or found work in a sheltered workshop.

Mobility Training

The mobility officer teaches suitable applicants to get about using a white cane or guide dog. Different types of cane denote the amount of training completed.

Gadgets

A braille clock or watch, needle-threading gadgets, adaptation knobs for cookers and guides for writing out pension or cheque books may be supplied. These, along with organised routines and familiar surroundings, may enable a blind person to be independent in his own home.

Education

Children with a visual handicap (whether registered or not) can be referred to the Advisory Teacher for the Blind from the Special Education Department of

238

Social Services. Education in normal schools may be possible if visual aids are supplied. There are also schools for the partially sighted and for the blind. Children usually attend these as weekly boarders.

Support

There are local and national support groups for blind adults and children, and a radio programme, 'In Touch'.

Royal National Institute for the Blind

The RNIB can supply information and aids and put written material on tapes or in Braille.

Braille

Many books are available in Braille (a system of raised dots which can be felt by the blind person). Braille clocks and typewriters are also available. A fairly high degree of intelligence is required to learn Braille and usually only the young blind master it. Moon is a simpler system of raised lettering more suitable for the elderly blind to learn. A 'talking book' (a tape recorder and taped books) may be loaned to the registered blind. Large-print books are available in most libraries for those who retain sufficient central vision to read them.

Low Vision Aids (see chapter 3)

These are dispensed by hospital opticians to a doctor's prescription.

Care of the Blind in the Eye Hospital

This includes those who are temporarily blind because of double padding or padding of their only seeing eye.

The nurse must know how to attend the blind patient so as to protect him from trauma without making him unnecessarily dependent upon her help. She should introduce herself by name before imparting other information. She should offer her arm for the blind person to hold, so that he can walk slightly behind her. The patient will sense from the movements she makes, any impending change of direction. He will feel more secure knowing that she will encounter any obstacle before he meets it. She should take his hand and place it on the back of a chair or on a bannister. The same applies to the chin rest of the slit lamp microscope, so that the patient can position himself correctly. Telling the patient the arrangement of food on his plate (meat at 6 o'clock, potatoes at 2 o'clock, etc.) may enable him to feed himself. Spectacles should be held by their ear pieces so that the eyes cannot be inadvertently poked as the glasses are put on.

GLOSSARY

Acute	having a short and relatively severe course
Anastomosis	a communication between two vessels, passages or organs
Anterior	situated in front of; the front or ventral surface of the body
Congenital	a condition present from birth regardless of its causation
Cryotherapy	the therapeutic use of cold
Dendritic	branching like a tree
Electrolysis	destruction by passage of an electric current (e.g., for permanent removal of eyelashes)
Epilation	the removal of hair (or eyelashes) by the roots
Extraocular	situated outside the eyeball
Fascia	a sheet or band of fibrous tissue such as lies deep to skin or invests muscles or organs of the body
Granulation tissue	a young vascularised connective tissue formed in the process of healing of ulcers and wounds
Granuloma	a tumour made up of granulation tissue
Hemianopia	defective vision or blindness involving half of the visual field
Homonymous hemianopia	blindness involving both right halves or both left halves of the visual field
Hypotony	low intraocular pressure
Hypoxia	low oxygen content
Infarction	an area of dead tissue due to local ischaemia
Ischaemia	local deficiency of blood usually due to obstruction of a blood vessel
Lateral	away from midline; to one side
Leucocoria	white pupil
Mydriatic	any drug that dilates the pupil
Myectomy	excision of a portion of muscle
Ophthalmoplegia	paralysis of the eye muscles

240

Palpating	examining the surface of the body by feeling it with hands or fingers
Papilla	the optic nerve head
Papilloedema	oedema of the optic nerve head
Paracentesis (bulbi)	puncture of the eyeball (usually anterior chamber)
Pathogen	any disease-producing micro-organism
Phakic	an eye with its crystalline lens still within it
Photocoagulation	coagulation of protein material by the controlled use of light rays
Phthisis bulbi	shrinkage of the eyeball
Prophylactic	a treatment that wards off disease
Prosthesis	an artificial substitute for a missing part (e.g., an artificial eye)
Recession	movement of a muscle towards its origin
Refraction	the art of determining refractive errors of the eye and their correction with glasses
Resection	excision (of part of a muscle)
Retinopathy	any non-inflammatory disease of the retina
Retinoscopy	an objective method for diagnosing and evaluating refractive errors of the eye by projecting a beam of light into the eye and observing movement of the light reflex seen in the pupil
Superior	situated above; the upper surface of an organ
Tachycardia	a very rapidly beating heart
Temporal	lateral (used of structures in the upper part of the head)
Tenotomy	the cutting of a tendon
Tentorium cerebelli	the part of the dura mater that forms a partition between the cerebrum and the cerebellum of the brain

FURTHER READING

Anatomy

Wolff, E., *Anatomy of the Eye and Orbit*. Revised Roger Warwick (Lewis, 1976, 7th edition)

Colour Atlas

Kritzinger, G.E., Wright, B.E., *A Colour Atlas of the Eye and Systemic Disease* (Wolfe Medical Publications Ltd., 1984)
Perkins, E.S., Hansell, P., *An Atlas of Diseases of the Eye* (Churchill Livingstone, 1971)

Contact Lenses

Ruben, M., *Contact Lens Practice: Visual, Therapeutic and Prosthetic.* (Bailliere Tindall, 1975)

General Ophthalmology

Trevor-Roper, P.D., *The Eye and its Disorders* (Blackwell 1974, 3rd edition)
Kennerley Bankes, J.L., *Clinical Ophthalmology* (Churchill Livingstone, 1983)
Phillips, C.I., *Basic Clinical Ophthalmology* (Pitman Books, 1984)
Galloway, N.R., *Common Eye Diseases and their Management* (Springer-Verlag, 1985)
Wybar, K.C., Kerr Muir, M., *Ophthalmology* (Bailliere Tindall, 1984, 3rd edition)
Newell, F.V., *Ophthalmology: Principles and Concepts* (C.V. Mosby Company, 1978, 4th edition)

Intraocular Lenses

Rosen, E.S., Haining, W.M., Arnott, E.J., (eds) *Intraocular Lens Implantation* (C.V. Mosby Company)

Nursing

Rooke, F.C.E., Rothwell, P.J., Woodhouse, D.F., *Ophthalmic Nursing. Its Practice and Management* (Churchill Livingstone, 1982)
Garland, P., *Ophthalmic Nursing* (Faber & Faber, London, 1975, 6th edition)
Smith, J.F., Nachazel, D.P., *Ophthalmologic Nursing* (Little Brown & Company, Boston, 1980)

Optics

Elkington, A.R., Frank, H.J., *Clinical Optics* (Blackwell Scientific Publications, Oxford, 1984)

Orthoptics

Cashell, G.T.W., Durran., I.M., *Handbook of Orthoptic Principles* (Churchill Livingstone, 1974, 3rd edition)

Physiology

Davson, H., *The Physiology of the Eye* (Churchill Livingstone, 1980, 4th edition)

Tropics

Rodger, F.C., *Eye Disease in the Tropics* (Churchill Livingstone, 1981)

Tumours

Bedford, M.A., *A Colour Atlas of Ocular Tumours* (Wolfe Medical Publications, 1979)

INDEX